ADVANCE PRAISE F(

"I'd been searching for resource   id
Alzheimer's disease and *Forget Me N*   If
you are facing the daunting task of caring for someone with Alzheimer's
disease, this book is an invaluable resource."

—Kathleen Lynch

"This book takes caregiving to another level. With *Forget Me Not*, I know
I can get through anything!"

—Michele Finn

"Author Debra Kostiw has created the definitive book to guide people
in caring for those with Alzheimer's disease. *Forget Me Not* offers all of
the tools you'll need to understand the disease and be in a position to
help the person you are caring for with their everyday living. I would
recommend this book to anyone who has a person in their life battling
this terrible disease."

—Matt Chandler, children's book author,
and son of an Alzheimer's sufferer

I

"Debra Kostiw's book, **Forget Me Not**, is spot on for anyone caring for a person with conditions like Alzheimer's. Kostiw takes the reader into the confusing and terrifying dementia landscape and presents ways to lovingly guide the affected person in his or her daily life. The data and protocols that she presents go far beyond what most health care professionals learn in school. A definite must have for all caregivers!"

—Sue LeDoux, RN

"**Forget Me Not** is an excellent resource that covers the major behaviors and care issues frequently seen in dementia. Each chapter begins with a concept that helps describe the reason for the behavior or care issue, followed by an easy-to-understand lesson that explains the context of the behavior. The concepts and lessons are followed by strategies and practical suggestions for interventions that can help caregivers avoid certain triggers or other well-intentioned approaches that might actually make the specific behavior or situation worse.

Caregivers who are well informed and supported usually feel less stressed and burdened by caregiving, and a wonderful resource like **Forget Me Not** provides the caregiver with much needed education about dementia while also offering practical solutions that any caregiver can easily implement. It is so important for caregivers to know that they are not alone and that there are effective resources and tools that can support them and their loved one. I encourage caregivers to keep a copy of **Forget Me Not** handy as they begin their caregiving journey.

The book is really well done and I am sure it will be very well received."

—Sharon A. Brangman, M.D., FACP, AGSF
Distinguished Service Professor
Chair, Department of Geriatrics
Director, Upstate Center of Excellence for Alzheimer's Disease
SUNY Upstate Medical University

"Wow! This is an absolute must read for any person caring for someone with dementia.

This is a very well written resource, simple, transparent, and right to the point. This needs to be in the hands of every life guidance and memory care community. As seasoned as I am, we forget. An excellent piece of literature with a purpose to educate!"

—Jeanette Cooper

"As a professional dealing with people with cognitive deficiencies I found this book extremely helpful. I discovered fresh ideas and practical techniques I could implement immediately! Kudos for **Forget Me Not**."

—Nicole Caruso

"*Forget Me Not* was a saving grace for me. I wish I had this expert resource in the beginning stages of my father-in-law's dementia. I found all the answers I needed and more. This beautifully written book is a complete guide to everything you need. I am a visual person and the illustrations really hit home. Debra shows you practical advice and offers help at every turned page. I'm going to keep several copies on hand to share with family and friends who are going through difficult times. It's the best gift you could ever give. Thank you Debra, for writing *Forget Me Not* and sharing your talents with the world!"

—Kim Burgess
Dedicated to Stanton Lee Burgess

"With the increase of dementia family members being cared for at home, this book is a must read to navigate through these trying times. Don't just read this book, implement it.

—Tami Kikta CNMT

"This book hits close to home as my mother is now experiencing some symptoms of dementia. This is a must have book for anyone that has a loved one dealing with this silent killer. It is an easy-to-follow book equipped with excellent illustrations to help the reader understand this disease. In addition, this book has real life questions and scenarios presented in ways to talk and deal with dementia so that your loved one will live their life with ease and comfort."

—Dr. Keith Tong, PhD DNM

"**Forget Me Not** provides an experienced professional's perspective on many of the challenges facing the families of Alzheimer's sufferers and offers practical and proven coping strategies and support resources to these families as they care their loved one during this difficult time."
—Katherine Liebner, Esq., elder law and estates attorney

"Debra Kostiw skillfully distills her decades of experience with this dreadful disease in **Forget Me Not**, an accessible guide for families and friends of loved ones suffering from Alzheimer's."
—Kevin Burke, attorney

"Every facility and every hospital should buy a copy of **Forget Me Not** for their employees."
—Alex Finn

"Debra pulls back the curtain to expose what's really happening for the person with dementia. This is an eye-opening experience showing you exactly what to do and more importantly what NOT to do!"
—Danny Lin

"I highly recommend **Forget Me Not** to everyone. I'm currently caring for my grandfather with dementia and this book has inspired me to be a better caregiver. It is so relatable and has helped me to understand what he's going through. Now we connect on a deeper level. For this I am truly grateful. 5 Stars!"

—Brittany McGhee

"**Forget Me Not** by Debra Kostiw is a must read for anyone who is struggling with and caring for a loved one who is suffering from dementia.... we don't know what we don't know.... sometimes we don't know what questions to ask.... this thorough and easy to understand book is an excellent resource offering information that is essential for caregivers to be successful."

—Tammy Jurkins OTR/L, CDP, CADDCT, CMDCP

"After reading the first few chapters of Debra's **Forget Me Not**, I can't wait for more! Already, I found it informative, innovative, and funny; also, it made me wonder whether I already have a favorite chapter or part of a chapter. These characteristics combined to make Debra's book thoroughly engrossing, and I will tell just about everyone I know the same!"

—Sandy Swanson

"Debbie, I wish I had your book when my mother was suffering with Alzheimer's in the 1990s. My father, sister and I would really have benefitted from it. A must read for anyone who has a relative or friend with dementia. Awesome!"

—Roberta Kerry

"Chock full of practical advice and eye-opening tips. This book, **Forget Me Not**, is the user manual [for dementia] you'll wish you had years ago. Highly recommended."

—Anonymous

"Wow! Debra outdid herself with such an easy reading style on such a difficult topic. These behavioral techniques are really eye opening. I wish I had this when I was assisting my grandmother and father through these challenges. Her simple tips are life changing!"

—Deanna Gutta, behavioral financial advisor

"Finally, a great resource for professionals and families starting to navigate the best care and response to individuals with dementia! This is a must read for anyone that touches and interacts with someone with memory issues. I found the illustrations in the guide, enhanced the message and lessons being offered."

—Laurie Bennett

"After reading this book. My belief is that it should be a training manual, for aides, nurses, family members, and home health care professionals. My mother has Alzheimer's, and I took care of her at home for 4 years. Now she is living in a memory care facility. My family is educated but they think if we love her enough, this will fix the Alzheimer's. Love does not fix Alzheimer's, education does. They do not understand Alzheimer's disease. They do not understand that her brain is dying. The same holds true with many aids and medical providers working in care facilities. I have had aids come into my home, they think if they yell loud enough, the person with dementia will understand them. People don't have enough knowledge or education about redirecting a person with Alzheimer's.

The illustrations are phenomenal because they made it simple to see and understand. With this book, **Forget Me Not** states exactly what to do for the person you love. The book talks about the concepts of the disease, the emotions associated with the disease process and covers sundowning, hallucinations, paranoia and more. **Forget Me Not** even showed me how I can talk so she'll hear me. It also trained me to listen more effectively so she can reply back to me. This book opened my eyes about how my mother was living in terror. Debra's book explained to me why my mother doesn't like to take a shower. I had no idea that it hurt so much and that it was so frightening for her. **Forget Me Not** showed me how to give her a shower with love.

I now know not to take things personally, and it has shown me how to do things differently and has helped me with what do with my own anger and frustration. This resource has helped me to love and treat my mother with respect.

Lastly Alzheimer's disease does not get better. It gets worse every day. I can't control it. But I can live with it, with this book. I know how to live with it now. This is why I believe this should be read by everyone that is touched with Alzheimer's or dementia."

—Carolyn Bean

"This is a $10K course in one book! I've taken many classes, and none have covered this topic as completely as *Forget Me Not*. Worth every penny."

—B.A.P

"Read it! Do it! Improve your life."

—Vincent Lam

"As an assistant nursing home administrator, I found this book to be helpful and encourage anyone that loves or works with memory care patients to use these tools. This book will have you thinking differently about communicating with memory care patients. *Forget Me Not* gives you the tools to use the basics. My favorite was the communication tools that show you how to set your loved ones up for communication victory, by reducing your stress and the anxiety of the memory care patient."

—Noah Sargent, nursing home administrator and radiology technologist

"In reading this book, a lot of actions I observed from my clients now make me understand why they were reacting to different situations in ways I would not expect. I am a licensed insurance agent specializing in Medicare. I now have a better understanding of why people with dementia act the way they do. Understanding why a person reacts to a situation allows the caregiver and the person receiving the care to get things completed. There are always actions that cause reactions. Understanding the actions can help control the reaction. This was a very fast read and I took notes for later reference.

Thank you for writing this book & bringing these concerns to my attention."

—Mark Waldman

"*Forget Me Not* by Debra Kostiw is a must-read for all of those who are in the battle of their lives. Caregiving is the hardest job you could ever tackle. Forget Me Not will be your best friend. No doctor or nurse can provide you with the skills or advice you need to get through your day. I personally feel that every doctor and every nurse should have this book memorized to help their patients and their caregiving family members."

—Judith R. Montgomery

"The chapter on behaviors was easy to follow, and understand, but most of all the concepts and practical advice came from someone who has experienced it and it hits home.

The everyday true-life examples that are given in the book are what a person with dementia and the caregiver struggle with. The solutions are simple, heartfelt, understandable and most of all manageable. I am a caregiver of both my mother and mother-in-law and this book is a go to for me personally. I reflected back on what I did, continue to do and how I need to change certain behaviors. This chapter for me affected me to the core.

Content was concise with a deep understanding of dementia. The examples were powerful as were the words that are used to describe and convey what needs to be communicated.

Debra is knowledgeable in the topic and is able to break down the struggles that are faced by the person with dementia and the caregiver. It is because of this that her book could be used as a guide for caregivers. It is a must read!"

—Rosa LaDelfa

"*Forget Me Not* provides excellent and very much needed information that is easy to understand. Great job!"

—TJ

"***Forget Me Not*** is a must-read for anyone who is caring for someone with Alzheimer's disease. The author outlines practical, helpful ideas to better connect with and care for your loved one. I found the exercises particularly applicable."
—Carl Bachman, grandson of an Alzheimer's sufferer

"Beautifully written by someone who understands not just medically but personally. Highly recommend."
—Debbie Vandewall

"Debra's many years of age-related mental decline is laid out clearly in this book. It is concise and provides clear guidance on the process and management of those affected by dementia and Alzheimer's. I highly recommend this book to any professional in this field."
—Garrett Fromme

"Just reading one chapter of **Forget Me Not** made me aware of the fragile condition that potentially affects each of us, let alone our older loved ones. But this writing on the subject of dementia/Alzheimers and its stigma, is very relatable in understanding this condition. I learned more than I ever knew just by this one opening chapter. The repetitive major points and mini-quizzes in the appropriate places are great reference points that can be easily recalled when dealing with difficult situations. Written from the point of view of the the affected individual, we are able to approach this condition with empathy just as Debra Kostiw explains it. A must-read for any caretaker or anyone with a friend or relative in cognitive decline in order to relate to this population with confidence and compassion."

—Lorna M. Davi, administrative assistant and fitness instructor

The #1 Alzheimer's and Dementia Guide
for Professional and Family Caregivers

FORGET

ME

NOT

Foreword by Dr. Sharon A. Brangman MD
Chief, Department of Geriatrics, SUNY Upstate Medical University
DEBRA KOSTIW
Illustrated by Olivia Kostiw

Forget Me Not: The #1 Alzheimer's and Dementia Guide
for Professional and Family Caregivers

Copyright © 2022 by Debra Kostiw

Illustrated by Olivia Kostiw

**Answers
About
Alzheimer's**

Answers About Alzheimer's

Rochester, New York

Printed in the United States of America

Hardcover ISBN: 978-1-959096-09-2
Paperback ISBN: 978-1-959096-10-8
eBook ISBN: 978-1-959096-11-5

DEDICATIONS

Dear Mom,

You were murdered twice. The first time was when Alzheimer's viciously attacked your brain and the second was the betrayal of your own son.

We were anxiously awaiting your homecoming in a few short days when we were robbed of the opportunity to make up for lost time. In your absence of two and a half years, had I known the torture you were enduring, I would have come to your rescue. Alas, I was too late. I deeply regret that I missed your subtle cries for help. I know that deep down you wanted to confide in me, and in some respects, you did, but mostly you were protecting me, as a great mother does for her child.

Your wish was to help your suicidal, murdering son. Again, as a great mother does. The Alzheimer's made it that much easier for them to physically, financially, and psychologically abuse you, take advantage of you, and ultimately steal your last breath from you.

I regret it took your death for me to clearly see the depth of your character, and the determined strong-willed human that you were. I now vividly see the depth of your strength, along with the love and tolerance you had for others. You were the most patient, loving, giving, soul. I am profoundly proud of the woman you were.

Mom, you deserved better. Way better! Especially at the end of your life. I wrote this book in your honor. You gave so much. Ultimately you gave your life. If I can help others to find their loved one deep beneath the damaged brain, then I have succeeded. I love you Mom, I miss you Mom.

Your loving daughter,

Debbie

Eleanor B. McGarigle 1928-2018

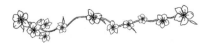

Many thanks to the illustrator, my dearest daughter Olivia,

With your spellbinding illustrations, *Forget Me Not* took on a whole other dimension. Thank you for creating the most beautiful graphics and bringing my vision to life. I am so honored and proud to be your mother. Your talents go far beyond your comprehension. It took me many, many years to find my strength and power. My hope is that you find your calling much earlier than I did and share with others, your infinite talents. The world needs you.

While this book may be my greatest achievement, you are my true pride and joy. I am so grateful that we were able to create this masterpiece together. I feel it has brought us even closer. I love you Olivia, more than anything.

If in the future I have a diagnosis of dementia, and I say hurtful, rude, nasty, painful, things to you, please file them away in your spam filter. I don't mean it. I love you, and at this moment, I apologize for any of my future behaviors, comments, or pain that I may cause you. I'm so sorry, I would never intentionally hurt you. I swear. I Love you.

Always,

Mom.

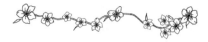

For Paul, my husband,

Thanks for holding the ladder steady for my climb to the top. Sometimes it was on shaky ground, but you always tightened your grasp when push came to shove. I hope your fingers aren't too bashed and bloody. The last couple of months you really came through. Making dinner every night, watching TV in the bedroom because my papers were scattered on every surface. Being silent when I snapped at you to be quiet because

I couldn't think. I appreciate the long silent car rides to and from the lake so I could work while you drove. Thank you for the seemingly endless budgets for every expense that I asked for, and so much more. Here's to another 30 years together. I can't wait to see what lies ahead.

Love,

Debra

CONTENTS

FOREWORD

Providing care to a person with Alzheimer's disease or a related dementia is among the most challenging of all the caregiving roles many of us will ever experience. One of the reasons for this may be because a person with dementia usually undergoes a simultaneous decline in both brain function and physical function that progresses over time and requires them to need more and more help just to get through the day. In addition, while caregivers are working so hard to meet their loved ones' needs, they may also meet resistance to their care, or encounter behaviors that only add to their efforts.

It usually falls on the caregiver to find creative solutions for behaviors that can be as varied as pacing and disrobing, or just finding the right activity to keep the person with dementia busy for a period of time. Caregiving can be a lonely and isolating experience at times, but some caregivers may not realize that there is no need to figure things out all on their own.

As director of the Center of Excellence for Alzheimer's Disease at SUNY Upstate Medical University, I have shared frustration with caregivers, since there are not many safe and effective medications that address the various behaviors that people with Alzheimer's disease or other dementias may experience.

However, the best interventions typically do not involve a pill, but rather, they require an understanding of the underlying disease process that cause the behaviors. There are lots of effective, non-pharmacologic approaches to behavior management that can be very helpful.

Forget Me Not is an excellent resource that covers the major behaviors and care issues frequently seen in dementia. Each chapter begins with a *concept* that helps describe the reason for the behavior or care issue, followed by an easy-to-understand *lesson* that explains the context of the behavior. The concepts and lessons are followed by strategies and practical suggestions for interventions that can help caregivers avoid certain triggers or other well-intentioned approaches that might actually make the specific behavior or situation worse.

Caregivers who are well informed and supported usually feel less stressed and burdened by caregiving, and a wonderful resource like *Forget Me Not* provides the caregiver with much needed education about dementia while also offering practical solutions that any caregiver can easily implement. It is so important for caregivers to know that they are not alone and that there are effective resources and tools that can support them and their loved one. I encourage caregivers to keep a copy of *Forget Me Not* handy as they begin their caregiving journey.

—Sharon A. Brangman, M.D.
Distinguished Service Professor
Chair, Department of Geriatrics
Director, Upstate Center of Excellence for Alzheimer's Disease
SUNY Upstate Medical University

August 26, 2022

*I'm trying my best. Be patient
with me.
Respond to my feelings, not my behavior.
I am scared, please protect me.
I need you.
I don't know what I should be doing.
I feel vulnerable, I don't feel safe.
I am lonely.
I'm trying to tell you, I need something.
Please listen, I want to be heard.*

Debra Kostiw

CHAPTER 1

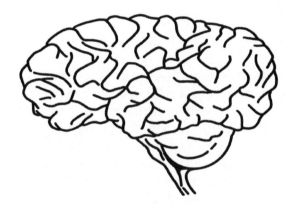

HOW TO TALK,
SO THEY'LL LISTEN

Concept

People with Alzheimer's or other dementias interpret language in distorted ways. Their brains don't process the information like we do. With a few tweaks, you can learn how to get your message across to them, and how to understand what they are trying to communicate to you. Everyone wants and needs to be heard. Everyone wants to be understood. Sadly, a person with dementia feels like no one is listening. They become invisible. Imagine what it would be like to no longer be able to convey your thoughts, wishes, or needs.

Lesson

Have you ever had an argument with someone who was drunk? How did that work out? It didn't, did it? Because one side was impaired cognitively. You can't win an argument with a drunk person, and you can't win an argument with a person who has cognitive decline. The brain cells have deteriorated, and their reasoning skills no longer exist. The part of the brain where negation and persuasion take place is damaged and can no longer function as it once did. It doesn't make sense to argue with a person with dementia. You will never win. Sorry.

As the disease progresses, communication will become more and more challenging. You must constantly be adapting your verbal and nonverbal skills to match their abilities. What works this minute may not work the next.

When two cognitively intact individuals have a conversation, it is a 50/50 exchange of information. When one of them has dementia, it is no longer an equal 50/50 exchange. How we communicate with others will influence their response, reaction, behavior, and the ability to perform tasks. Conveying messages is key to our self-expression through our thoughts and feelings. We share our wishes and desires through communication. Interacting with others is how we form relationships and how we exhibit our personalities and character. This chapter will be the foundation for all the following chapters, and it will be referred to often. You will want to revisit it several times.

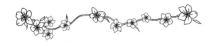

Communicating with a person with dementia is challenging enough. Providing them with as many opportunities for success will benefit everyone.

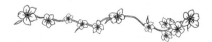

Set Them Up for Victory!

Messages are sent, and messages are received. At least that's the goal. It's up to us to make sure the message that is sent is simple enough to penetrate the damaged brain, get to the desired destination, and be understood. There's a lot of steps involved with the processing of information. The message sent will have to travel through billions of healthy neurons, taking multiple detours, avoiding the dead and damaged ones, to make its destination. That's not an easy task for the cognitively impaired individual. Providing people with as many opportunities for successful communication is going to benefit both the sender and the receiver.

Start with these communication basics.

- Have their attention.
- Give them time to process and reply.
- Provide a quiet environment.
- Have only one person speak at a time.
- Let them know you are listening.
- Use short, simple sentences.
- Speak slowly.

- Speak clearly.
- Use signs instead of words.
- Use gestures instead of words.
- Help them find a word.
- Offer a guess.

Combining these simple strategies will set them up for communication victory. First and foremost, make sure you have their attention. It may take them several minutes to realize that you are in the room. Remain in one spot until they are able to focus on you. Get down to their eye level. If you are towering over them, they will feel intimidated. They need to see your face. Our eyes show emotion and build trust. It's also harder for them to hear your voice when you're towering from above. After speaking, pause and wait for a response. Those with Alzheimer's or dementia need much more processing time. It can take them up to twenty seconds or more to respond to you. Twenty seconds is a really long time to wait for a response.

Perhaps there are too many people in the room or too much background noise. Distractions from ambient noise can disrupt the flow of communication. People with dementia cannot differentiate your voice from background noises. Creating a quieter environment will greatly improve the chances for receiving messages. This will be covered in depth when we get to the chapter, "The Horror They See That You Don't." Use shorter, simpler sentences, speaking slowly and clearly. Focus on the key words. As the disease progresses, you will rely on gestures and pictures more often. Eventually, the person may not understand the spoken word. If English is their second language, chances are they will revert back to their native language and no longer understand English. If they are struggling to find a word, you can or offer a guess, but don't jump in to help too quickly; give them enough time to spit it out. If you attempt to help too early, they may get frustrated or angry. You will be breaking their concentration, and they will have to start the process all over again. We will expand on this later in the chapter.

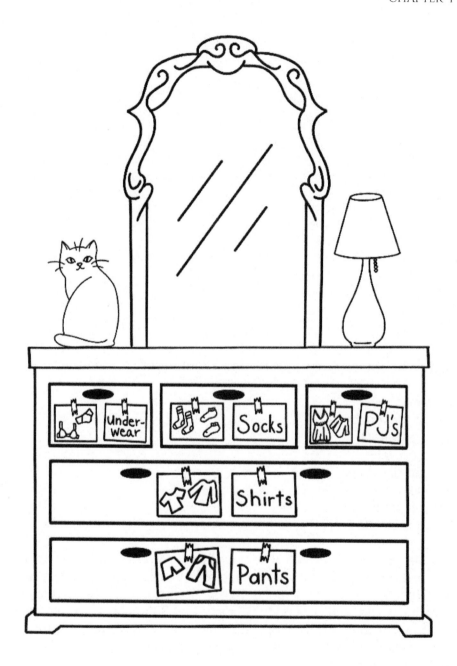

Play by Play

Using Gestures

Come Sit	Pat the seat of a chair.
Brush Teeth	Act out the motion of brushing your teeth. (modeling)
Hungry?	Pat your stomach or act out putting food into your mouth.
Tired/Sleep	Place your hands by your face and close eyes; make a snoring noise.

Other Important Communication Techniques

- Smile
- Gentle touch
- Eye contact
- Eye level
- Body language
- Facial expressions
- Stay in one spot
- Tone of voice

People with dementia will read your facial expressions and body language. It tells a lot about you. It can also influence how the person with neuro-deficiencies will respond. Believe it or not, only 7% of communication is verbal. 55% is body language and 38% is facial expressions. That means that over 90% of communication is nonverbal. People will react to how the information is delivered before they process what was said. Fascinating.

What Do These Facial Expressions
Say to You?

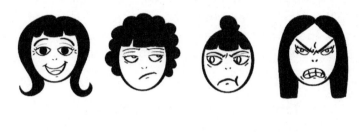

_____   _____   _____   _____

What Do These Body Languages Say to You?

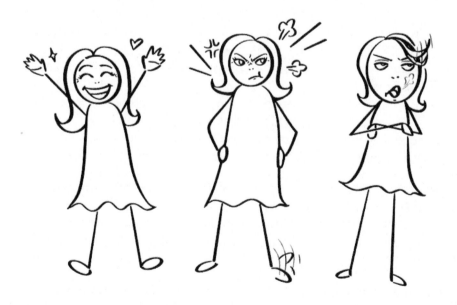

I'm_____   I'm_____   I'm_____

Would you jump in the shower for figure number two or three? No. You don't trust her. You don't like her. She's mean! If you want the person you are working with to be relaxed and happy, then that is exactly what your facial expression and body language must say to them. Check yourself! And if you must, fake it. If you're having a bad day, they can sense that. When they don't understand your words (and even when they do), they are responding and reacting to your facial expressions and body language. It's not about you, it's about them. The receiver.

Do Not...And I Mean Never!

- Use baby talk.
- Quiz them.
- Correct them.
- Argue with them.
- Hurry or rush them.
- Talk about them while they are present. (Never whisper in the other room; you'll be sorry.)

Imagine you are involved in a conversation with people who are obviously intellectually superior to you. You have no idea what the conversation is about. Then suddenly someone asks you a question. All eyes turn on you and they're waiting for your reply. How do you feel? Be honest. Anxious? Frustrated? Stupid? Challenged? Angry? Belittled? People with dementia feel this way **all the time.** I am going to say that one more time. People with dementia **feel this way all the time.** They know that they are not getting it. In most cases the person with dementia is aware that their brain is not working the way it should. This is terrifying for them.

People with dementia WANT to please you. They WANT to answer you. They WANT to perform the task. If they could, they would. But they cannot due to the damaged brain. We will dive much deeper into this in the "Validate and Captivate" chapter, but you're not ready for that just yet. We must lay the foundation first.

Stop quizzing. Do not ask them who the people are in photographs or pictures. This will only frustrate them. Don't say, "Come on, Mom, you knew who this was yesterday." How do you think that's going to make her feel? Mom will think, *Why don't I know that? What's wrong with me? Should I know that person?* How scary would that be for her? Remember, they are living in the past. The person with dementia may be living during their life of ages 15 to 24. So older photos are better for reminiscing rather than more current photos of grandchildren.

Do not baby talk to an adult; it makes them feel like a child and they are not a child. Everyone is important. This is about dignity. They are adults and must be respected as such. Remember, these people have a brain disorder. They have lived a full, rich life. They have had important jobs, raised families, built a lifetime of experiences. Be respectful with your tone and refrain from addressing them like a toddler. Someone once told me, "This is the hardest age to adjust to." Another said, and I quote, "It didn't take me eighty years to get stupid." To age successfully takes great strides. With our help, we can assure the aging process remains dignified.

Executive functioning is the ability to perform tasks in a particular order. Early on in the disease process our executive- functions skills begin to diminish. The cognitive load, or the difference between a single task and a series of steps, puts a tremendous strain on our executive functioning. Simplify and slowdown, which brings us to the next point.

Tick tock. You can't turn back the hands of time, but you can give a person with dementia all the time they need. Most people will eventually answer you. Provide them with enough time to process what you said. The compromised brain needs more time for the information to travel to the correct part of the brain, retrieve the information, and then for the response to travel back. If needed, try using a different word. Providing shorter, simpler sentences will help the processing time for them. Think of moving in slow motion.

Play by Play

As the disease progresses and communication becomes more challenging, adapting our language and adjusting to their abilities will prove critical for understanding the wishes and needs of the person with dementia. It's important to keep the interactions positive. In upcoming chapters, we will get very specific on how to keep the communication positive.

As noted, during the various stages of cognitive decline, the focus on how we communicate needs to shift. Spotlight the key word to get the message through. During which, we must adapt to the ever-changing abilities of the person as the brain deteriorates. The sentences will eventually be reduced to one or two words. Refrain from asking questions that rely on memory and begin using gestures and signs. You will be amazed at how many gestures you can use to communicate with your loved one.

Our YouTube channel is filled with more tips for communication. Tune in at Answers About Alzheimer's.

Say "This"- Not "That"		
Too Long	**Early-Mid Stage**	**Later Stage**
"What do you want for lunch today when Michelle comes over later?"	"You hungry?" OR "Let's go eat."	"Eat" (Sign to eat.)
"Don't go outside. It's cold out and you don't have your shoes on."	"Stay with me."	(Sign to come.)
"Which outfit do you want to wear today?"	"This or that?" (Show them two choices)	"Here." OR "Put this on."
"It's time to take a shower and get ready to go to the doctor."	"Let's wash up." OR "Spa day."	"Wash up."
"Here you go, it's time to take your pills.	"Here you go."	"Take these."
Go put your pajamas on and brush your teeth. It's time to go to bed."	"Rest now." "Time to retire." "Let's brush our teeth."	"Here." (Hand them pajamas.) "Put this on." "Brush." (Hand them the toothbrush.)
"Hey, Mom, would you like to go for a walk? It's so nice outside today."	"Let's walk."	"Come."

Play by Play

For most of us, speaking and having conversations with others comes naturally. It's not a skill that you typically stop and contemplate before doing, unless you're a public speaker on a stage. We don't spend time choosing each and every word. They just flow out of our mouths. The problem with this is our dialogue, and the words we choose, are often perceived as confrontational to a person with cognitive disabilities. It's not necessarily hard to make a conscious effort to use different words, but it does take some practice. Because we talk on auto-pilot, we need to slow down and think of how our words are interpreted by the receiver. The win-win here is when you slow down and choose your words more carefully, this in turn gives the person with dementia more time to process the conversation. While awkward for us, it provides them with more opportunity for success. The following chart is a reference of words that should be avoided as much as possible. The trigger words can have a negative connotation.

Trigger words can be perceived as disrespectful for the person with neuro-deficiencies. Instead, refer to the column on the right, offering a more appropriate choice. Refining your choice of words will reward you and your loved one with more positive verbal exchanges.

Trigger Words vs Safe Words

Trigger Words	Safe Words
You can't!	Let's try this.
No!	Do it this way.
Diaper	Brief
	Absorbent underwear
	Absorbent undergarment
	Protective pants

Trigger Words	Safe Words
Change Diaper	Clean up, wash up.
	Let's get comfortable.
	Let's adjust your brief.
	Let's switch your underwear.
Bib	Dining Scarf
	Smock
	Shield
	Clothing smock
	Shirt cover
	Apron
Change Clothes	Attire
	Get gussied up
	Fashion show
	Dress up
You Have to...	Will you help me?
Don't! / Stop!	Try it this way.
	Come with me.
	Do it this way.
Good-bye	See you soon.
	I'll be right back.

Trigger Words	Safe Words
Bedtime	Retire for the evening Rest Sleep
Go to the doctor.	Let's go for a ride.
Shower	Spa day Wash up Freshen up
Take your meds.	Here. The doctor said … We don't want to end up in the hospital.
Come here!	Will you help me? Let's go this way.
Bathroom	Ladies/Men's room Take them to the bathroom. Bathroom break Toilet

Are They in Pain?

When communication is hindered by cognitive decline, individuals may not be able to express that they are in pain. Assessing and diagnosing pain in those with dementia presents many challenges. Nonverbal cues indicating that the person may be in pain include:

- Irregular breathing
- Teeth grinding
- Guarding
- Crying
- Wincing
- Tense-ridged body posture
- Fidgeting
- Rocking
- Agitation
- Frightened facial expression
- Furrowed brow
- Squinting eyes tightly shut
- Tightly grasping bedding or handrails

If you suspect that the person you are caring for is in pain, do not delay. Contact the doctor, hospice, or palliative care professionals immediately. When in doubt, call 911 or head to the emergency room. Remain calm and provide soothing activities such as music, storytelling, gentle massage, or stroking. After pain medications are given, note the time the dose was administered and monitor closely for recurrence of pain.

Language Deficit Definitions

Anomia: Unable to retrieve the correct word or proper name of an item.

- Example: Hand me that thingamajig. Where is the, the, the...

Paraphrasia: A common language barrier when the sentences get all mixed up or the message appears meaningless to the receiver. Can also be garbled, made up words that have no meaning.

- Example: I oak tree this cool car in the teeth. Or globestesternes, Farralingthack.

Agnosia: When a person with dementia cannot recognize or identify an ordinary object or has trouble with facial recognition.

- Example: A woman held up a banana and asked, "What do I do with this?" Although she recognized the item as something familiar, she did not know what its purpose was. When she was told, "You eat it," she smiled and opened the banana and ate it.

Neologism: Using similar words that mean the same thing but have an altered vocabulary.

- Examples:
    - Folded Food=taco
    - Closet box=drawer
    - Red sauce and bread= toast and jelly
    - Toe shirt=socks
    - Big white bowl=toilet
    - Tinsel paper=foil
    - Plastic notepad=iPhone
    - Christmas circle=wreath
    - Seed holder=bird feeder
    - Wrist clock=watch
    - Flat hotdog=bologna

If you would like a complete list of definitions and descriptions on language deficits go to www.AnswersAboutAlz.org for a free PDF download.

Exercise

Fix these sentences

"Hey, George, let's go to the Seafood Shack and get a fish fry for dinner tonight. We can bring it home if you want."

_____

_____

"Hey, Ellie, why don't you go get dressed, and we'll go to Denny's for lunch today? It's your favorite."

_____

_____

"How are you feeling today? Do you still have a headache? Maybe we should call the doctor."

_____

_____

"Come on, we have to go to the store and then stop at the post office before they close."

_____

_____

How can you sign to someone it's "time"?

_____

_____

How can you sign to someone to "come" to you?

_____

_____

How could you sign to someone to "eat"?

_____

_____

How could you sign to someone to go for a "walk"?

_____

_____

List six nonverbal cues that someone may be in pain.

1. _____

2. _____

3. _____

4. _____

5. _____

6. _____

Change These Trigger Words to Safe Words

"Hey, don't go outside!"

_____

"Stop, that's hot!"

_____

"Time to go to bed."

_____

"Do you have to go to the bathroom?"

_____

"It's time to take a shower."

_____

"You can't cook anymore."

_____

"I think you need your diaper changed."

_____

"Put your bib on; it's time to eat."

_____

"No! Stop! You have to put your underwear on first."

Reflection

Keep it short and simple; give them enough time. Don't rush them. Remember your facial expressions and body language. Smile. Use a soothing voice. Be kind; they are trying. Choose your words carefully; don't instigate an argument by using the wrong words.

If you would like a complete list of definitions and descriptions on language deficits go to www.AnswersAboutAlz.org for a free PDF download.

CHAPTER 2

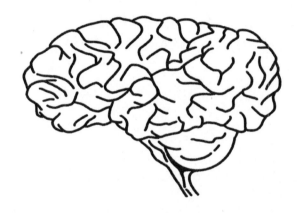

ADVICE FOR BEHAVIORS YOU'D BE CRAZY NOT TO TAKE

Concept

Let's get one thing straight right off the bat. The sooner you understand this the better.

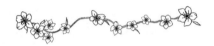

THEY'RE NOT GIVING YOU A HARD TIME. THEY'RE HAVING A HARD TIME!

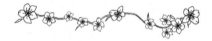

The way we behave is a form of communication. When a person with cognitive disabilities has a disruptive behavior, it is a sign to you that they want or need something. Their perception of their environment is unpleasant to them. It feels incredibly frustrating not to be able to communicate what you need.

A behavior is the way in which a person **acts in response** to a particular situation, the environment, a person, or stimulus. The key word is **response**. They are responding to something. In this chapter we will learn how we can help predict and control the responses from a person with dementia through their perception. Have you run across any of the following behaviors?

Aggression	Paranoia
Wandering	Sexual disinhibition
Repeating	Toileting
Hallucinations	Bathing

Eating   Screaming

Removing clothing   Shadowing

Anger   Accusations\stealing

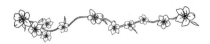

Dealing with behaviors can be exhausting for everyone involved. When we discover what the need is, we can eliminate the behavior.

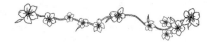

Lesson

Behavior- The way in which a person acts in response to a particular situation, the environment, a person, or a stimulus. They aren't just behaving badly or acting out for no reason. They are responding to something or someone that is having a negative effect on them. Think about that. Knowing they are having a reaction to something means we can avoid the action that causes them to react in a way that we want to avoid. Behaviors are a direct correlation to one of the following:

Physical (pain, uncomfortable   Too much/too little stimulation
clothing)
                                       Fear
Unfamiliar environment
                                       Frustration
Communication

If you are caring for someone who is exhibiting unpleasant behaviors, you need to become a detective. Search for clues and investigate to identify what they need. Going forward, you'll discover how to conquer the most frustrating behaviors. It's all here for you.

You can learn so much more about managing challenging behaviors by visiting www.AnswersAboutAlz.org.

We have loads of fun on our YouTube channel, Answers About Alzheimer's. Subscribe today!

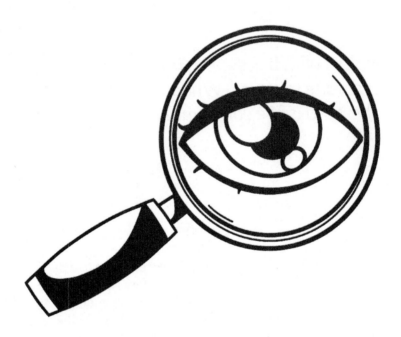

What makes you angry and frustrated?
What pushes your buttons?

They are not being stubborn. They are not being difficult. They are not being lazy. THEY DON'T HAVE ALL THEIR BRAIN CELLS. What causes a behavior? People act out when they feel **powerless or vulnerable.** People with dementia feel this way all the time! Because of the brain damage, they cannot communicate their wishes, or when they do, it comes out in a way they did not intend, like an insult, or words that don't make sense. They act out because they need something. As the cognitively intact caretaker, it is up to us to be the detective. We must look for the clues and try our best to determine what they need. Discovery equals peace. Preempt the behavior by intercepting **before** it happens. You can do this!

What causes behaviors? Think about what gets you frustrated? What makes you angry? What are your breaking points? When do you lash out to others?

Causes can include:

Hot\cold

Pain

Vision and hearing impairments

Confusion

Afraid/fearful

Frustration

Too much stimulation

Not enough stimulation

Unfamiliar surroundings

Too much noise

Tasks are too complicated

Searching for something or someone

Feeling stuck

Don't know what to do next

The need to toilet

Uncomfortable clothing

Unfamiliar people

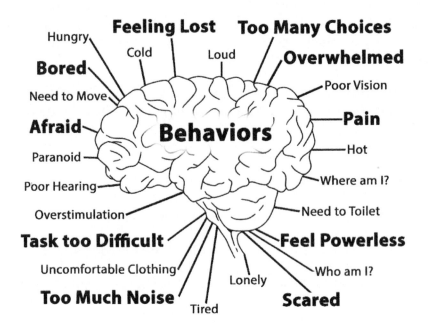

Feeling Lost
Hungry
Cold
Loud
Too Many Choices
Overwhelmed
Bored
Poor Vision
Need to Move
Afraid
Pain
Paranoid
Hot
Poor Hearing
Where am I?
Overstimulation
Need to Toilet
Behaviors
Task too Difficult
Feel Powerless
Uncomfortable Clothing
Who am I?
Lonely
Too Much Noise
Tired
Scared

Dos and Don'ts

Your Approach

How you interact with someone who is upset will either make the situation better or it will make it worse. Referring to the chapters, "How To Talk So They'll Listen" and "Validate and Captivate," be very attuned to your facial expressions, body language, and tone of voice. Try not to react. Respond to their emotions and feelings, not the behavior.

- Watch your facial expression.
- Watch your body language.
- Watch your tone of voice.
- Use a gentle touch.
- Respect personal space/boundaries.

- Reassure them they are safe.
- Let them know you are listening.
- Approach from the front or dominate side.
- Focus on their feelings, not their actions.
- Reduce noise levels.
- Ask how you can help.
- Validate their reality.
- Change the subject.
- Redirect to an activity.
- Let it go.
- Try humor. (We all need to laugh more.)

Their emotions and feelings are real. Do not dismiss or reject how the person feels. Let them know you are listening. When they are reassured that they are being listened to, they will feel validated. The person with dementia needs to feel a sense of control. Give them their power back. Use phrases like:

- "I'll help you."
- "I've got you."
- "I'm here for you."
- "Let's look together."
- "Don't worry."
- "It's okay."
- "You are safe."
- "Show me."
- "I'm so sorry."
- "Can I help?"
- "We've got this."

The following scenario is a true story that took place in a memory care community.

The Behavior

It was getting late in the evening and the aides had to get the residents ready for bed. This particular aide approached Victor, took him by the hand, and said, "Come on, it's time to put your PJs on and go to bed." She led him by the hand to his room and asked him to get undressed and put on his pajamas. He said, "No." She asked again; again he said, "No." At this point, the aide reached towards his chest to unbutton his shirt. Victor smacked her hand away. The aide was getting agitated and continued to insist that he change his clothes. She attempted again, and again he smacked her hand away saying, "Don't touch me." She then reached for his trousers. He had enough! At that moment, he shoved her into the wall. A couple seconds later, five or six people ran into his room and tackled him. The story to the family went something like this. "Your father is uncooperative, combative, and violent. You're going to have to hire a private aide 24/7 to watch him." (Not true. The staff at the community did not have proper training.)

The Solution

The aides were told to get everyone in the community ready for bed. The aide approached Victor and said to him with a big smile, "Hi Victor. Everyone is **retiring** for the evening. How about we go and get your **night clothes** on? Would that be okay with you?" They walked together to Victor's room and when they arrived, she asked him to put on his **night clothes**. He refused. She smiled and laid his night clothes out on the bed and then left the room for a while. The aide returned later to see if Victor had changed into his pajamas.

The Difference

This time the aide used adult words like "**retire**" and "**night clothes**" instead of childlike words like "PJs" and "bedtime." She smiled and did not lead him to his room by the hand like a toddler. She also asked Victor if it was okay with him, giving him a choice. When he refused, she stayed calm and gave him space. When it was clear that he did not want to change his clothes, she let it go. There was no reason why he must change into his evening attire. When she attempted to help him get undressed, he may have interpreted that as an inappropriate sexual advance. This action may have made him extremely uncomfortable. There is no safety reason to insist that Victor change into his pajamas, be flexible. Let this one go.

The story to the family from the community should have gone more like this: "I wanted to let you know that your father got a little upset last night. The aide was trying to get him to go to bed. He was not cooperative, and he refused. The aide pushed back, and I think he may have misunderstood her intentions. He felt like she was forcing herself on his personal space. He did push her, she is okay, I've had a meeting with her, and we've done some additional sensitivity training. But I just wanted to let you know why your dad is still in his day attire from yesterday."

Communities should NEVER blame the patient. They HAVE BRAIN DAMAGE! Come on, You can't BLAME someone for their actions/reactions when they have a brain disease!

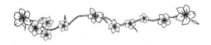

Respond to the Emotion
Behind the Behavior

How to Respond

Try giving them something to hold, reassure them. Play music, sing songs, hum, or try nature sounds. Comfort them. Ask how you can help. Listen... They want to be heard! Turn tapping into an activity. Tapping is a form of communication. They are trying to communicate with you, they need something. Have the person tap to the beat of music or turn to another tactile activity such as arranging faux flowers or sorting things. (Refer to "How to Keep 'em Busy in Ten Seconds or Less.") The person with dementia may be trying to let you know they need to retreat to a quieter setting.

Fixations and Obsessions

Some people with dementia will get stuck or fixated on something. They fuss and fidget. Once they start, they can't stop. It's like they're obsessed. Cutting or tearing paper, checking the locks, rearranging the cupboards, making the bed again and again. These behaviors can be irritating to say the least, but let's take a look at this exasperating behavior from a different angle. In upcoming chapters, we go to great lengths to learn how to distract a person with dementia into an activity. Fixation is an activity! Just because you don't perceive it to be purposeful, to them it is relevant and meaningful. This is a win. Celebrate!

If the person is self-entertaining, and they are safe, the best approach is to just let them be. Is it bothering them or you? Actions that drive you up a wall are self-soothing to them.

Rummaging through drawers or closets can keep a person busy for hours, but they may leave you with a big mess to clean up later. Try creating a rummage box. Put various items together that would create interest or spark long-term memories for them. Consider the types of things they are already focusing on or rummaging through. For example, if a man used to tinker in the garage or the basement, you could place items in an old cardboard box labeled "Stuff." If Mom loved jewelry, get a substantial jewelry box and load it up with shiny, glittery costume jewelry, gaudy pins, and maybe an old photo of her parents. The point here is to turn this behavior into a more meaningful and personalized experience.

Another problematic fixation that I've come across frequently in my career, is an obsession over finances and bank statements. Constant worry about money and the loss of control over their finances is very distressing for people with dementia. If this has been a problem, you can create a feeling of security by giving them a little pocket money or fake money to carry in their wallet or purse. Make up some bogus financial documents. Prepare fake bank statements, checkbooks with figures written in them, IRA and investment paperwork. Mix in some other mock bills that say PAID on them and add some junk mail into the mix. Try to create a hefty stack of papers for them to rummage through. Arrange the papers as they would have in the past. Where did they keep these documents? How were they stored and arranged? Recreate their past experiences.

Having lost control over so many aspects of their life is a source of pain for them. This is a way to give them some of that power back.

Fixations and obsessive behaviors relieve anxiety and distress. This person needs something to do; they are bored. Their brain is saying, "What am I supposed to be doing? I should be doing something." They feel out of control. Inadequate. Reassure them that they are important and you're glad they are there to help you. They need to be productive and feel important.

Shadowing and Repeating

Some people with cognitive disabilities will follow you everywhere. You can't get a second to yourself. When someone follows you around and around, and you just can't shake them, they are feeling very insecure. They are afraid and clinging to you for comfort. This person feels that they should be doing something, but they don't know what it is. They cannot initiate. Be reassuring and comforting to them. Try giving them a stuffed animal, fidget toy, or a squeeze ball to hang on to. This person does not feel safe and secure. Can you imagine how frightening that must be for them? To feel unsafe?

The constant repeating of questions can drive even the most patient caregiver to the edge of a cliff. Try to remember that this repetitious behavior will not last forever. And yes, you need to answer them again and again. Your person with dementia is feeling insecure. It's not about the question; they are seeking comfort and security.

When they are asking you the same question over and over, try having them write the answer on a white board or a note and refer them to it, or ask the question back to them. The part of the brain responsible for storing our most recent memories has been damaged. Never say things like, "You just asked me that," or "I just told you." Try asking them to tell you a story or divert to a task to "help you." Perhaps sorting buttons or matching socks- lots and lots of socks. Ask them what they are feeling. If they keep asking what day it is, they may be feeling like they are forgetting something important. They may be trying to ask for help with something but cannot figure out how to communicate those wishes to you.

In the movie *Groundhog Day*, Bill Murray is about driven to insanity while he experiences the same day over and over. Have you ever reached your breaking point because your person with dementia is experiencing these annoying symptoms? These repetitive behaviors can be verbal or nonverbal. They may state the same word or phrase repeatedly. Or they may be yelling or tapping their hands. It's enough to drive you nuts. Remember that all communication has meaning behind it. As the cognitively intact, we must take the time to discover what the need is behind the behavior.

When should we let them be, and ignore the behavior, and when should we be concerned?

Causes for Repetition

- Over or under stimulated
- Feeling insecure
- Fearful
- Uncomfortable positioning
- Uncomfortable temperature
- Looking for something or someone
- Basic needs
  - Thirsty
  - Hungry
  - Need to toilet
- Trying to communicate wishes
- Feeling stuck
- Pain
- Unfamiliar surroundings
- The need for an activity
- Attempting to self-soothe
- Need for purpose

Pacing

I'm the kind of person who is always on the move. I've been that way my whole life. In the past my friends called me a spaz. Although I'm not a fan of that terminology, it is true that I don't like to sit still for extended periods of time, so I guess that would be an accurate analogy. For instance, when I'm having dinner at a restaurant, I find that after about an hour, I'm ready to get moving. My brain and my body have had enough.

Have you ever seen an animal at the zoo pacing back and forth in their cage? This animal is coping with stress by disengaging from its environment. The animal is attempting to relieve feelings of anxiety. Humans will also pace, resulting from a stimulus or lack of. When a person with neuro-deficiencies has a restless behavior like pacing, we must look beyond the restlessness and evaluate what the need is behind the behavior. They may be requiring a more comforting environment or seeking out familiar surroundings. If it's not possible to go for a long walk outside because the person is in a locked memory care unit, poor weather conditions, or the time of day, just let them be. If they are safe, let them pace. Is this behavior more of a problem for you, or for them?

There are many things to consider when identifying possible pacing triggers:

- They just need to move
- Environment is confusing
- Feeling lost
- Looking for something or someone
- Basic needs, toileting, hunger, thirst
- Boredom
- The need for engagement
- The need to exert energy

Stealing and Accusations

Most people with dementia will go through a period where they believe that others are stealing from them. Obviously, this can be difficult to overcome, but we can certainly take some steps to help. First and foremost, make sure they know you are listening. "Well, if that happened, I promise I'll do my best to get to the bottom of it."

- Don't take it personally.
- Stay calm.

- Let them express worries.
- Say you're sorry.
- Ask them to help you find it.
- Try to get them to show you their secret hiding places (also helpful for future accusations).
- Who do they trust?

Try phrases like, "I thought I saw it a little while ago," or "I think it was put away for safekeeping."

A solution may be to have duplicate items that look similar. Many women will hide their purse under their pillow at night for safekeeping.

"I'm going home!" Out the door they go!

There can be several reasons why a person with dementia is asking to go home. Home is a place where we feel comfortable and safe. It's where we release all our tensions from the outside world. We are protected there. Let's review that a person with dementia is often living between the ages of fifteen and twenty-four years old. So, when they say, "I want to go home," they may be thinking of where they lived during that age range. It will be helpful if you can get that information in case they pull a disappearing act; you might find them at that address. The person suffering from the brain damage is overwhelmed and cannot make sense of their environment or where they are, even if they have been living in that home for the last forty-three years. Can you even begin to imagine how it must feel to not know where you are, and want to go home? Unfamiliar surroundings or people can cause the brain to create a feeling of frustration and fear. They don't feel safe.

Never say, "You are home. You've lived here for forty years." Or "You moved here a year ago." This will only make them more frustrated, angry, confused, and/or scared. Remember to put yourself in their reality, their dimension. Rule out that their basic needs are being met. Do they need to toilet? Are they hungry or are they overwhelmed by their environment? Something or someone is making them feel uneasy. What is it that they are reacting to?

So, what do we do? There are some techniques to keep a person from exit seeking. Most people won't leave without shoes or a coat. Most women won't leave without their purses. So, we can remove or hide these trigger items. You can try getting ready to go and then divert to a favorite activity. You can also try saying something like the following sentences and then blend into a favorite activity. Oh, I can't wait to turn you on to the "Validate and Captivate" chapter!

"We can't go today; they are painting."

"Let's put it on the calendar for tomorrow."

"Your husband asked if you would help me with this puzzle."

"Your (mom, brother or sister) called and asked if you would help me with these tasks until they get here."

Ask them questions about the place they are missing.

"Tell me about your home; describe it to me."

"What are your favorite things to do at home?"

"Tell me about how you spent the holidays."

"That's a great idea. We'll go as soon as I get this laundry done."

Making it sound like it was their idea gives them power! If worse comes to worse, get in the car and go for a drive. Maybe stop for a treat. How can you make them WANT to stay in that environment?

Hallucinations and Paranoia

A hallucination is when a person sees something that does not exist. It is vivid, detailed, and can involve all the senses. Hallucinations most commonly involve seeing or hearing children or other people, animals, or insects. 13-20% of those with dementia will hallucinate. People are more apt to hallucinate if they are sleep deprived or have altered sleep patterns. (Common in Sundowning.) In most cases, hallucinations don't seem to bother the person with dementia. They may talk about seeing people in their home or outside, but mostly the hallucinations don't upset them. If this is the case, let them explain to you what they are seeing. Validate their reality, and do not correct them. Remember, we never argue with a person with a degenerative condition. Be a source of comfort for them. Reassure them that they are safe, and that you will protect them. Show them your confidence in protecting them. Try to redirect to an activity using the techniques below and, in the chapter, "These Diversion Techniques Can Change Your Life."

Illusions are a false interpretation of existing situations. They often involve people or animals and are most common in Lewy body dementia. With an illusion, people may see faces in a pattern or interpret their surroundings incorrectly. A perfect example would be where someone interprets a shadow on the wall as an intruder or an animal. An illusion is when our eyes play tricks on us. Most people are not bothered by these visions, in which case it is best to simply acknowledge and overlook it.

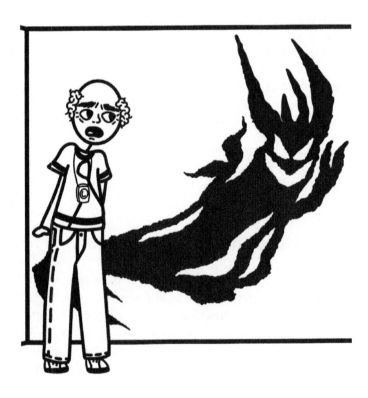

Delusions are very strong false beliefs. The person with dementia will firmly believe and argue until the end of time that this false belief is true. DO NOT let them suck you into an argument. You must agree with them and let them have this one. A delusion is based on feelings. Acknowledge their feelings, apologize, and promise them you'll do better. These are not to be confused with hallucinogenic visions. A delusion is a made-up story. A false story that they firmly believe to be true. The most common delusion for the person with dementia is that someone is cheating on them or stole something from them. They are very suspicious of others. They may believe that someone is trying to poison them, or they may believe they are an astronaut and just came back from outer space. The best way to try to overcome delusions is to go with the flow. Cheating is a tough one. Their feelings are hurt. You can say something like, "I can see why you would think that" or, "That makes sense." "I love you and I'm so sorry I made you feel this way. That's awful. Can I make it up to you?" We are going to cover more of this topic later on.

With these types of statements, you are not accepting any wrongdoing or admitting guilt, but you are reacting to their emotions. Are you getting this?

Delirium usually has a sudden onset of symptoms. Typically, within hours or days. Symptoms include hallucinations, anxiety, and a heightened state of confusion among others. Delirium is a **temporary** mental state and is **reversible**. Episodes of delirium are caused by an infection, dehydration, drugs, alcohol, and more. People with cognitive disabilities whose dementia symptoms spike rapidly may have an infection causing the delirium. A UTI or urinary tract infection can bring on these sudden symptoms and is reversible with a course of antibiotics.

Dealing with hallucinations, delusions, and delirium can be particularly challenging. It is vital that you do not tell them that they are hallucinating. This is also not something you should disagree with or argue about. Validate their feelings. Let them know that you believe them. Make sure they feel heard. Remember, you cannot argue with someone with dementia. They have brain damage. Their reasoning skills no longer exist. If the visions are frightening or upsetting to them, and all your attempts to divert and redirect fail, it may be time to have the neurologist intervene and prescribe antipsychotic or other drugs as a last resort. We will get into more detail on responses when we get to the chapter on "Validate and Captivate." Again, remain calm, reassure them. Put on your poker face. Use words like:

- It's okay.
- I'll protect you.
- I'm here.
- I'm your bodyguard.
- I'll save the day.
- I don't see it, but that doesn't mean you don't.
- I'll take care of it, don't worry.

Remember to respond to their emotions not the behavior.

Sexuality

We are social creatures. We all yearn for intimate, meaningful relationships with others. Just because we age doesn't mean that we lose our desire to feel connected. Dementia does not diminish the need to be physically close to another individual. This need transcends the loss of memory and the ability to understand the nature of relationships. Intimacy and closeness are not just the act of having sexual intercourse. It's so much more than that. It's about emotional pleasure. Intimacy and pleasure include touching, kissing, flirting, hugging, hand holding, and cuddling. The desire and need to express ourselves sexually dose not disappear with age or with dementia. Sex continues to be an important part of our lives. More than 40 percent of couples age eighty to ninety-one living at home, where one or both partners have dementia, are sexually active. Sex has many health benefits as well. It is great exercise physically, boosts our self-esteem, reduces anxiety, improves physical and mental health, and releases endorphins.

Sex, intimacy, and self-expression later in life is important to our self-confidence and well-being. Do not discriminate against our seniors who are sexually active. They are not "cute" or "adorable." That's your bias and it's ageism! Get over it.

Scenario

A move to senior living was recommended for Edith after her husband had passed away. She had Alzheimer's and it was not safe to live on her own. One evening in her confused state, Edith wandered into the wrong room. She accidentally climbed into bed with Mike, another resident living down the hall from her. In Edith's mind, this was her normal behavior. This was her routine for the past forty years. Within Mike's presence, she might be looking for comfort, protection, or she might just want to get warm and cozy. Edith didn't recognize this man as a stranger. In fact, she found comfort with him. She felt safe.

When the staff discovered that Edith had accidentally gone into the wrong room and climbed into bed with her neighbor, they gently reassured Edith that Mike looked a lot like her husband. They asked her, "Please come with me," and calmly escorted her back to her room. The staff was careful not to embarrass or shame her during the exchange. Edith may have been looking for comfort or perhaps she was lonely. Try offering her a stuffed animal or a doll to hold to provide that soothing feeling. This behavior will eventually pass as her progressive brain damage moves on to the next area of her brain. (We do not tell Edith that her husband has passed away.)

Edith and Mike should not be the next topic of conversation spreading throughout the care setting, involving both staff and residents. Edith and Mike's interaction was a private matter. It's not gossip. This is about respect. Please don't make me go there. That's going to be another book! Just decided!

Mistaken Identity, Masturbation, and Disrobing in Public

The limbic system is where the sexual part of our brain is located. When this part of the brain is viciously attacked by dementia, it can distort or even heighten our sexual desires. Dementia warps our reality from knowing what appropriate conduct is and what is not. Manners are no longer understood by the individual and social filters have disappeared.

(What's my excuse? Haha.)

Common inappropriate behaviors can include masturbating or disrobing in public, pinching, grabbing, or making sexual comments to medical staff and family members.

When a person with cognitive disabilities needs assistance with bathing, toileting, and dressing, these activities can be misinterpreted as a sexual message. We absolutely must keep in mind that these actions do not reflect who the person is. They are not a pervert. This behavior is due to the deteriorating brain. The effected brain has lost the ability to control impulses.

Those with dementia lack regular physical touch and are often lonely, miss the companionship of others, and are looking for comfort, but cannot express what the real emotional need is. They are trying to let you know that they lack a feeling of inclusion, and this is the only way they can express it. They are apologizing to you, through me, right now. Forgive them.

Mistaken Identity

Because the person with dementia is lost in time and living in the past, they may not recognize their loved ones. It is common for a parent to mistake their children for a spouse or their brother or sister. At this point, they may not even know that they had children. They may look at their elderly spouse and think that person is their mother or grandmother. They do not recognize the person because they are looking for a younger version of that person.

A perfect story of mistaken identity was when Diane went over to visit her father. When she walked into his bedroom to help him get up and ready for his day, he was excited to see his wife. He immediately made a sexual comment and tried to grab her and pull her into bed with him. At first, the daughter was horrified, but she remained calm. Diane told her father that she wanted to freshen up, and she'd be right back. Diane left the room and proceeded to change her appearance. She put on items that she knew her mother would never wear. Diane stuffed her hair up inside a baseball cap and put on a graphic tee shirt. She waited several minutes, and then reapproached her father as if it were an entirely new day. As she re-entered the room, she announced loud and clear, "Hi Dad! It's Diane. Your daughter. I'm so glad to see you." With this greeting, it gave Dad the opportunity to recognize her as someone other than his wife.

Best Practices

When a family member is assisting with personal hygiene activities like bathing, this can be confusing for the person with a declining memory. They may interpret bathing as a sexual act. Wearing scrubs to look like a medical professional may help.

If sexual behavior is aggressive in nature, stay calm and project confidence. Be firm but refrain from scolding or shaming. Don't point or shake your finger at them. Responding in a calm, professional manner will give you better results. Use their formal name, Mr. or Mrs.\Sir or Ma'am rather than their first name. This response could also be applied in situations involving pinching or grabbing.

Helpful Phrases:

- "No. Respect my personal space."
- "Stop that."
- "That is not appropriate."
- "You're crossing the line."
- "I'm setting boundaries."
- "That's going to stop. Now."
- "I will not tolerate that."

Disrobing and Masturbation in Public Spaces

When we are dealing with public disrobing or masturbation, the best approach is not to draw attention to the behavior. Disrobing in public could mean several things. The clothing they are wearing might be uncomfortable, they may think it's time for a shower, they may need to toilet, or maybe they're too hot. It might not have anything to do with sexuality.

When a person is fondling themselves in public, the first thing to remember is that they don't realize what being "in public" means. The person with dementia lacks social cognition and loses the ability to control impulses. The reason for self-stimulation could simply be that they want to gratify themselves, or it could mean they need to toilet, or they need to be involved in an activity, their clothing could be uncomfortable, etc. You should be seeing a pattern here. Always rule out basic personal needs first.

Our Response

Try to cover the person with a blanket and let them know this is not the time or the place. Be gentle. Escort the person to a private area and let them be. Remember, sexuality is part of our basic instincts. Never shame or embarrass the person.

Racist Comments and Slurs

Seniors who have Alzheimer's or other related dementias have no social filter. They no longer understand what is appropriate or inappropriate, resulting from the brain damage. They can't help it. When these very hurtful statements are voiced, it can be extremely difficult to remember that this is out-of-character for the person and is related to the disease. They have a very limited vocabulary, and they are not consciously choosing the words that come out. Language is one of the first affected areas of the brain.

Currently, we are in a culturally diverse landscape. But in years past, this was not the case. It is important to remember that the person with dementia is living between the ages of fourteen and twenty-five years old. Imagine what their reality was during that time of their life. They grew up in a much less diverse community setting. They had life experiences and cultural practices that influenced what the person believes. We cannot be sure one way or the other if they are a racist. They are simply not used to interacting with people from other ethnic backgrounds. They do not understand the feelings of others. They are fearful and anxious and don't have the social skills or brain power to rationalize these feelings. Ideally, no one should ever have to deal with these types of remarks, especially at work, but understanding how the disease process affects the brain can provide some comfort and clarity. Take the following into consideration:

- How did their childhood shape their beliefs?
- What are your own unconscious biases?
- Do you own them?
- Do you acknowledge your own thoughts about cultural differences?
- Was racism part of your upbringing?
- What were your experiences?
- Could past experiences that have shaped your life come up for you when you have Alzheimer's or dementia?

These unseemly comments are very painful, to say the least. I personally cannot imagine how awful and hurtful this would be, and yes, some people are racist. However, it is not effective for us to react. It solves nothing either way. Try to remain calm. There is no benefit to believing the person truly is racist. As hard as it may be, it is important that we don't react to these statements. We must be firm without scolding or lecturing. Having some counteractive ways of responding will be helpful for everyone involved. (Refer to the chart on safe words.)

We have a support group for you on Facebook. Search: Groups, Answers About Aging & Alzheimer's.

Maybe start out with…"You're smarter than that." Then follow up with:

- "It's nice to see people from other cultures coming together."
- "Come on, give me a chance."
- "That wasn't very nice."
- "Please, let's be polite."
- "Let's be courteous of each other."
- "That is not very helpful."
- "Please be kind."
- "Can we please get along?"
- "Let's put our best foot forward."
- "My wish is that we become friends."

After making your best effort to diffuse this very unpleasant exchange, try to divert to an activity or another topic of conversation. If the situation erupts, then remove yourself from the area. Try your best not to react.

Check out our website **www.AnswersAboutAlz.org** and our **YouTube channel Answers About Alzheimer's for more information and tips on these difficult topics.**

If you would like Debra to come and train your staff, reach out via email at Debra@AnswersAboutAlz.org.

Hateful Comments

They say the darndest things! If only it were that easy! Rude, crude and unrefined. Do you remember that old saying? The deterioration of the brain results in a physical attack on our personality traits and our characteristic patterns. We spend a lifetime building and cultivating our reputation, only to be reduced to being held captive within our own mind. But as the disease takes over, we are taken prisoner, no longer able to "think before we speak." When we can no longer filter out or control these negative comments, it can destroy our relationships in just a few short exchanges. The fluctuation in personality becomes our loved one's burden.

Rude - Offensive, Bad Manners

Crude - Lack Tact or Taste

Unrefined - Lack Moral or Social Cultivation

When a person with dementia lashes out and says things so hurtful that it penetrates like venom, we must remember that they don't have inhibitory control.

Computers have a spam filter that detects unsolicited, unwanted, and virus-infected messages from penetrating your sensitive equipment. You've got to protect your sensitive equipment. Turn on your spam filter and see a different perspective. Choose to take that ugly comment and file it away. It means nothing. There was no malicious intent behind it, so don't let it torture you. File it under spam and move forward. The more legitimate message they are trying to convey to you is buried far beneath the nasty comment they just slung at you.

Your objective is to find the true source behind the comment. Most likely they are afraid or nervous about something. The frontal lobe region of the brain that forms our character and personality is under attack. They can't help it. The dementia has their character held hostage.

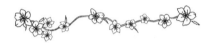

You're not being attacked.
Their brain is under attack.

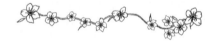

Dementia has no boundaries.

Communication in the Last Stages of Dementia

Vocalizations or a repetitive movement may be the only way they have left to communicate. Can you imagine how frightening it would be if you could no longer communicate your desires and needs? Never assume that they do not understand you or that they cannot hear you. There is a story in the last chapter about Janet the potter, and how she was completely unresponsive. But then when a piece of her beloved pottery was placed in her hands, she awoke one last time. Finding joy and meaning for the person and letting them know that you are not ignoring them will bring them comfort. In many cases, they just want to know that a loving person is close by. Those in the later stages may only be able to communicate by:

- Yelling "Help" or "Help me." Or other single words or phrases.
- Moaning/Groaning
- Rocking
- Tapping

Do not allow staff at a skilled nursing facility, hospital, or any community setting to tell you that the woman down at the end of the hall screaming, "Help me, help me," is fine. She is NOT fine! This person is in distress. Ignoring a person's basic needs at the end of their life is abuse. We've all heard it, and we must never hear it again. It haunts me. Give this person the attention they deserve.

Play by Play

A concerned daughter called my office, and she was very upset about her father. He was living in a memory care, and the facility kept calling her to say that he was not doing well. The memory care unit said that her dad was paranoid and thought people were out to get him. The community was unsuccessful trying to calm him down. They advised the daughter that she would have to hire a 24/7 private duty aide or put him on some heavy medications. Neither of these options seemed doable for her. I told the daughter that her father was feeling out of control, and he felt that he was in danger. Poor soul!! "I have a solution for you," I said. "We will send a large male caregiver, and he will tell your dad that he is his personal bodyguard. The bodyguard will tell him, 'I am here to protect you, and if you don't see me, it's because I am in disguise.'" Problem solved!

How do you handle when Mom comes to you and says someone stole her watch?

- "Well, if this happened, we will get to the bottom of it."
- "Let's look for your watch together."
- "I'm so sorry this happened to you."
- "I'm sure we will find it."
- "I will help you."
- "Don't worry."
- "It's okay."
- Offer a blanket or stuffed animal to hold. "It will bring you good luck."

- "It was put away for safekeeping, but I can't remember where we put it."
- "It's at the jeweler's, getting a new battery."

Problem

Mrs. Harkness was obsessing about the pile of leaves down by the street. She was constantly saying to her husband that the leaves had been there for days, and she was very upset that the town had not come to pick them up yet. The repetitiveness was driving her husband crazy.

Solution

Say, "The town hasn't picked up the leaves? (Validation.) I know! They haven't picked up mine either! (Match her frustration.) You have every right to be upset! (Give her power.) I'll call and find out what's going on." (Solution.) Pick up the phone and pretend to make a phone call and have a conversation. Hang up and say to Mrs. Harkness, "Oh my gosh, the town said that they were so sorry. The truck broke down and they will come as soon as possible." Close the curtains.

- Validate her concerns.
- Match her frustration/anger.
- Give her power.
- Solve her problem.

*I'm acting out because I'm desperate
for you to listen to me!*

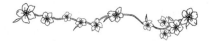

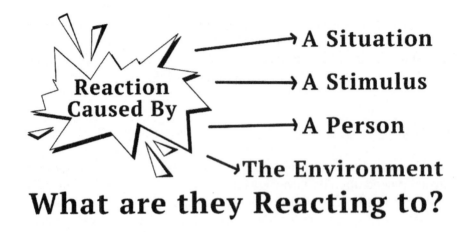

What are they Reacting to?

They're not giving you a hard time.
They're having a hard time.

Behavior/Action	Solution/Rule Out
Toileting Urge to go no longer perceived by the brain Urinating in odd places Cannot find bathroom	Past toileting habits, simplify clothing, use signs, 2-hour toilet reminders, shame/embarrassment.
Eating Eat raw food Brain no longer signals hunger Only wants sweets	Dry mouth, poor fitting dentures, dental issues, problems swallowing, boost or ensure protein drinks, can't see contrasting food on plate, quiet dining environment, move to finger foods.
Dressing Wearing clothing inappropriate for weather Disrobing in public Wearing the same clothing every day	Too hot/cold, too many choices, lay out clothes in proper order, allow enough time, have several of similar outfits, remove out of season clothing, let it go.
Bathing Purpose of bathing forgotten Refusing	BATHING MAY BE PAINFUL! Room too cold, fear of bathing, cannot make sense of color contrast of room, bathing preferences, let them wash their own face. DO NOT POUR WATER OVER SOMEONE'S HEAD!
Sleeping Sleeping during the day Awake during the night	Not enough exercise, temperature of room, napping too long, door and blanket preferences, limit caffeine, melatonin.
Wandering/Pacing Want to go home Let them pace if safe	Feel lost, can't make sense of the environment, reduce noise, camouflage doors, remove trigger items, shoes, purse, coat, door alarms, bed alarms, searching for something or someone.
Repetitive Actions Vocalizations, Moaning, Tapping Repetitive action may be necessary to move onto the next step	Only way to communicate, need to tell you something, fear, need to toilet, anxiety, NEED FOR ATTENTION! LONELY! BORED!
Sundowning Heightened confusion, anxiety, disorientation later in the day and through the night	Tired, increased shadows create anxiety, more exercise, close curtains, lower expectations, have activities ready.
Sexual Disinhibition Disrobing Masturbation in public	No longer understands inappropriate behavior, do not overreact, remain calm, be reassuring but direct, have a blanket to cover the person, lead to a private area.

Exercise

Janet says she wants to go home now. What are three ideas you could try to reassure her? (Do not tell her she is home.)

1. _____

2. _____

3. _____

When Ellie expresses that she wants to go home, what are three feelings that she may be experiencing?

1. _____

2. _____

3. _____

Helen comes to you, and she is frantic. Helen is clearly upset about something. She is crying and is yelling that her purse is missing. Someone stole it! What actions can you take to help Helen? (Don't tell her it didn't happen-validate/acknowledge her feelings.)

_____

_____

_____

It's evening and time for bed. Brian is wide awake. Brian used to work C-shift his entire adult life. He seems anxious and keeps pacing. What should you do? (Don't tell him he is retired and doesn't work anymore.)

_____

_____

_____

James seems particularly agitated today and is just not himself. He is being uncooperative and combative when approached. What are some things we can try to rule out? What questions can we ask James?

_____

_____

._____

Reflection

You're really dealing with emotions not behaviors. Behaviors can be minimized and even prevented. When a person acts out, it is because they want or need something. They act out using behaviors out of desperation. Look. Listen, Learn. It's all they have left.

CHAPTER 3

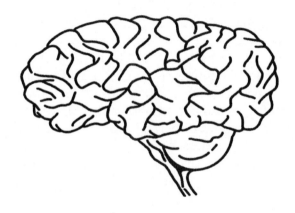

VALIDATE AND CAPTIVATE
VERSUS
CORRECT AND PERSUADE

Concept

If you correct a person with dementia, you make them feel stupid and inadequate. If you attempt to persuade them, you will only make them get more defensive. However, if you VALIDATE their feelings, it defuses those feelings, and then you can CAPTIVATE their attention.

Lesson

Okay, let's get one thing straight. If I haven't made it crystal clear already, they have brain damage. You can't argue or persuade a person with brain damage. It's like arguing with someone who is drunk or on drugs. Can you win an argument with them? No. Why not? Because they are using a brain that is under the influence. A person with dementia is working with a brain that has atrophy, which means it has shrunk. The cells are dying. Their brain cells are not capable of making the connections like our brain cells do. Arguing, disagreeing, or trying to prove a point will never work. I repeat, it will never work. In fact, you will make the situation worse. If you try to convince or push a point with someone with dementia, they will feel even **stronger** about it. It will backfire on you. People who have cognitive deterioration are strongly attached to their fears and opinions. Accept the fact that you're not going to convince them to change their mind. The sooner you do this, the easier both of your lives will be.

The closer we are in the relationship, such as a parent, spouse, sibling, or a child, the more comfortable we are criticizing or correcting them. This corrective behavior is very destructive to a relationship. Especially if one is cognitively declining. Being told we are wrong is not only insulting and belittling, but it affects our sense of self-esteem. It makes us angry. When have you ever been corrected by someone and felt happy or empowered by it? Did you jump up and down with excitement when you were convinced you were wrong? No one wants to be proven wrong.

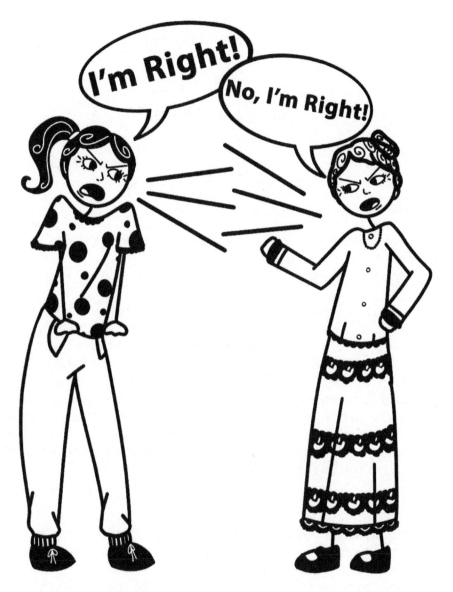

If you're the kind of person who needs to always be right, (as I tend to be sometimes) then you're in for real trouble. This concept will be extremely difficult for you. Vow to make a change in your habits. Learn to give it up. Let it go. Remove your ego. Do it now, for everyone's sake. Be the hero. It's the difference between peace and harmony or resentment and frustration. Not to mention keeping the relationship out of turmoil. Don't let being right wreck your relationship. Dementia not only deteriorates brains, but it also deteriorates relationships! Again, be the hero. You can do it!

Correcting and Persuading

Play by Play

WRONG WAY

- "Dad, you can't drive anymore, remember? The doctor said so."
- "Mom, I just told you that. Oh my God."
- "Stop pestering me!"

That doesn't feel good or comforting. It makes them feel stupid, angry, and confused. Responding like that is going to get you more behaviors and more push back! That's what that'll get you. More trouble! You can't correct, and you can't persuade someone with dementia. Again, they have cognitive degeneration. You will never win them over. Not even with hard facts. You can't rationalize with them. They no longer have the capacity to be persuaded. That part of their brain just doesn't work anymore. So don't waste your breath. Instead, take a breath. Correcting and persuading will not work. EVER! (Refer to the Safe Words Chart in the "How to Talk So They'll Listen" chapter.)

RIGHT WAY

- "Dad, I'm sorry. The car is in the repair shop, waiting for parts. As soon as it's ready, we'll go for a ride." (This is a lie, of course, but it makes them feel good and calms them down.)
- "Mom, I'm going to write the answer on the board for you. Can you help me write it down? Then let's go do your favorite activity." Validate then captivate. Move into an activity.

So how can we get through to them? Because, the hard truth is, we cannot correct them, and we cannot persuade them. If you tell someone who is afraid, **not** to be afraid, it only makes the situation worse. Instead, acknowledge their feelings behind the fear. Let them know you understand, even if you don't share that fear. Their fear is real! It's real to them. Pretend it's real for you too. Put on your best acting performance.

If you tell a person who is hallucinating or delusional that what they see isn't real, what do you think their response will be? Do you think they will just believe you, and their terrifying hallucinations will just magically disappear? Hell no.

If you tell them nothing is there or that they are hallucinating, you are going to make it worse. Because now you've made them feel like they have to **prove** it to you. You have just challenged a person with dementia. What happens when you're challenged? **You fight back.** You get defensive. Don't be the one to say something that creates a challenge. Don't try to prove a point and start an argument. **When a person with dementia is told it is okay to feel something, it encourages them to stop fighting to justify it.** It's okay to feel a certain way. Remember, they can't help it.

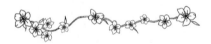

When we're told, "It's okay to be afraid," we are often less afraid.

When we are told, "It's okay to be suspicious," we are often less suspicious.

When we are told, "It's okay to be angry," we are often less angry.

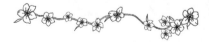

Persuading means to pick flaws in the others' thinking. That's pretty much all they have now, flaws in their thinking. So, stop picking. You're just picking a fight. Persuasion is a form of communication and communication is not strong for them anymore. Remember to respond to their emotions and feelings. Validate, don't correct. It's no longer an even 50/50 dialogue. The cells in that part of the brain are dead.

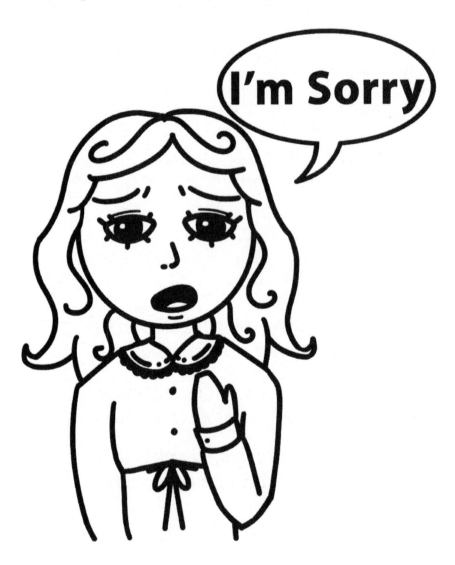

Validate and Captivate

It must be done in that order. Validate first, then captivate. (Refer to the "Keep 'em Busy" chapter.) Give them the best gift ever! Just because we don't agree with them doesn't mean we can't acknowledge and validate their point of view. **We can sway them indirectly, by siding WITH them.** Think of the peace of mind they would get if you did that for them. It's okay if we don't share the same feelings or emotions, but it's not okay to dismiss the way the person with dementia is feeling or what they are experiencing. Whether it's reality or not, it's how they feel. It's their experience. Acknowledge and validate their feelings behind the fear, anger, or hallucination. Let them know you understand, even if you don't. Lie!

Do they have an enemy? Is someone out to get them? Well, team up! Join the battle! Tell them you've got their back and you'll fight like hell! "Don't worry, I've never lost a battle yet! We'll get through it together!" Play at their game. Play like you did when you were a kid, with a vivid imagination. Be the actor you've always wanted to be. Get on stage and put on your best performance! The person with dementia is your audience. Validate whatever they are experiencing and pledge to resolve it, come hell or high water! Whatever it takes!

Make sure they know they are being heard by repeating what they said to you, back to them.

Mom says- "She stole my purse!"

You say it back to her- "She stole your purse?"

Dad says- "Those men were in my room again last night!"

You say it back to him- "Those men were back again?"

VALIDATE FIRST

ALWAYS ACKNOWLEDGE THE EMOTION/FEELING FIRST! These important statements confirm that they are being heard. It helps them feel comfort and promotes a sense of self-dignity and satisfaction.

- "I'm sorry your _____ is missing."
- "That must be stressful for you."
- "That has happened to me before; it's an awful feeling."
- "Oh no, that's terrible!"
- "I'm sorry you're upset."
- "I believe you."
- "You're right."
- "I understand."
- "I agree."
- "That makes sense."
- "I'm so sorry; this is hard stuff."
- "I see how upsetting this is for you."
- "It's totally understandable that you feel this way."
- "I care. Tell me more."
- "I don't know what to say, but I'm here for you."
- "That would bug me too."

Validation

Acknowledge the possibility that they are correct. For example, the statement, "That makes sense," leaves them feeling empowered without admitting guilt. They need to know that you've heard them. It's hard to argue with someone who agrees with you. Agree, don't disagree. Recall in the "How to Talk So They'll Listen" chapter, be aware of your body language, use a gentle touch, and watch your tone of voice. Revisit that chapter if necessary. It's chock full of crucial information. Are you starting to see how everything comes together?

Next Captivate

Join their team. Have their back. Solve their problem. Use your fairy dust if you must! This is when you find the humor. It's time for therapeutic lying. Yes, it's okay to lie to a person who is upset or to avoid an argument that you won't win anyway, so, why bother? You're actually being kind by stretching the truth.

- "Tell me what it looks like."
- "I'll help you look."
- "If she did take it, we'll get to the bottom of it; don't worry."
- "She moved it for safekeeping, but I can't remember where she said she put it."
- "Let's look together."
- "I've already spoken to the police, and they've promised to take care of it."
- "Tell me what you see."
- "Tell me what's happening."
- "Can you describe it to me, so I understand better?"
- "Oh, I saw on the news, they caught that guy."
- "I chased them away."
- "You are so smart; we can figure this out."
- "Together we can."
- "We'll get through it together."
- "I'll help you."
- "I love you; I want to help."
- "It's okay…"

Those with dementia have far less control over their feelings and emotions. They have trouble expressing them, and when they do, they may come out in odd or exaggerated ways. When a person with dementia has trouble expressing their emotions, they may overreact because they are unable to self-soothe or rationalize with themselves. It's okay if they feel a certain way. Remember, they can't help it.

When we are told, "It's okay to be afraid," we are often less afraid.

When we are told, "It's okay to be suspicious," we are often less suspicious.

When we are told, "It's okay to be angry," we are often less angry.

Life is unpredictable.
Things don't always go
the way we planned.
Lower those expectations.

Exercise

When you correct a person with dementia you make them feel _____.

Who is wrong? (Circle one)

Me   Them

A person with dementia cannot reason. Therefore, we will never try to_____them.

I need to make my loved one feel _____.

Always_____ first, _____ second.

The first step is to validate their feelings/emotions. Write five sentences to validate someone's feelings/emotions.

1. _____

2. _____

3. _____

4. _____

5. _____

Repeat what they said back_____.

Write five sentences to captivate them.

1. _____

2. _____

3. _____

4. _____

5. _____

Reflection

People with neuro-deficiencies feel like they lack control and have no choices, resulting in negative feelings and poor self-esteem, which creates the perfect storm for behaviors. Correcting and persuading should be avoided at all costs. The plan is to validate and captivate. Give them back their power. You got this!

For more tips on validation techniques visit www.AnswersAboutAlz.org.

We have some great roll-playing techniques on YouTube, Answers About Alzheimer's.

CHAPTER 4

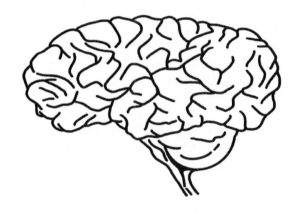

HOW TO KEEP 'EM BUSY
IN TEN SECONDS OR LESS

Concept

They are in the state of static! Learn how to bring them out of the static!

Lesson

Activities define us. They help us express who we are as individuals and promote dignity. A sense of purpose is directly related to our self-worth. Activities consist of everything we do, whether it relates to our work, personal life, relationships, spiritual, or are recreational. They offer a sense of direction and inclusion. Everyone needs to feel included. A meaningful or purposeful activity can be as simple as brushing our teeth or shaving our legs or face. It can be working in an office or going to a family picnic or attending religious services. Activities are how we remain connected; they make us feel important. They give us a reason to get up in the morning.

Without activities, we are in a state of static. We are just taking up space. Those within this stage of brain damage are stuck. Sometimes this is mistaken by the caregiver as being lazy, but really, they are no longer able to initiate or start an activity. However, they will usually be able to accomplish a task if it's not too complicated, they are given enough time, and have the right trigger. In many cases, modeling or showing them what you want them to do is helpful. (Refer to the communication, "How to Talk, So They'll Listen" chapter.) The brain will remember skills that were learned a long time ago. For example, if you take an electric razor, hand-over-hand and put it up to his face and start the shaving motion for him, it may trigger the long-term memory, and he will become unstuck, out of the static, and begin shaving.

It is vital to make sure that the task we are asking is not overwhelming or they will shut down and refuse. Ahhhh, yes, the refusal! Now you're getting it. Feeling overwhelmed or the task is too difficult is the number one reason why they refuse or freeze up. The key here is to introduce one step at a time, slowly.

Consider This

We must modify the difficulty of the task to accommodate the abilities of the person. This can change from day-to-day or even minute-to-minute. BE FLEXIBLE AND LOWER **YOUR** EXPECTATIONS. Usually, people with dementia are more successful and able to perform tasks earlier in the day. As the day goes on and they get tired, the span of attention is diminished. Give them enough time to understand what is being asked of them. This is very important. If they don't understand what you want from them, how would they possibly be able to do it? Make sure the undertaking is not too long. This may frustrate them and with frustration comes behaviors. Decide when it is time to step in and help, or take over and finish it for them, or simply end the activity.

If it's decided that it's time to end the activity prematurely, don't make it sound like it's time to quit because they couldn't do it. Make sure it's not perceived as a failure on their part. This is devastating to their self-esteem. Simply say, "That's enough for today," "That was great," "Fantastic, all done," "Well done," or "Perfect." This is a balancing act and may also change from day-to-day or minute-to-minute.

Limit distractions to help them focus on the task. Going back to the chapter "The Horror They See That You Don't," consider what is going on in the background. Are there too many distractions? Too many people in the room? The person with dementia cannot dismiss these environmental distractions, and they will not be able to perform the task. Let us also be mindful that the activity is age appropriate. For example, a simple puzzle. This means that it is an adult puzzle with fewer, larger pieces and not one that was designed and manufactured for infants or toddlers with the red knobs on them.

Factors to Consider for a Successful Activity

- Level of abilities
- Time of day
- Length of the activity
- Quiet environment
- Task is meaningful to the person

- Age appropriate

People are happy when they have a purpose. People who have dementia and are happy will have fewer behavioral problems. That said, we can affirm that if we can help maintain the abilities of the person and give them enough time to complete a task, they will feel a sense of accomplishment, thus promoting self-esteem. Remembering that the focus needs to be on having fun or having a purpose, the emphasis is NOT on finishing a particular task, it is also NOT about completing the entire activity.

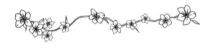

Process Vs. End Product
Fun Vs. Frustration
Purpose Vs. Perfection

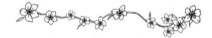

Set Them Up for Victory!

- Have fewer choices.
- Simplify the task.
- Minimize distractions.
- Mornings are usually best.
- Help initiate if needed.
- Slow down.
- Don't correct. (Say, "That's an interesting way to do that.")
- Be encouraging/smile.
- Jump in if needed.
- Quit while you're ahead. * (That's my favorite.)

Play by Play

Imagine this. Someone is going to assign you a task. You are asked to assemble something. You are then escorted into a large airplane hangar, and before you lie all the dismantled parts of an entire airplane. You are handed an instruction book and told "Go ahead, put this together." "Start here." That is what a person with dementia feels like when you ask them to do a task that is too complicated for them. They see all those airplane parts. They see all those steps. They just don't know where to begin, so they shut down. It's too overwhelming! When introducing an activity, be sure to add each step, one at a time, rather than having it all out at once.

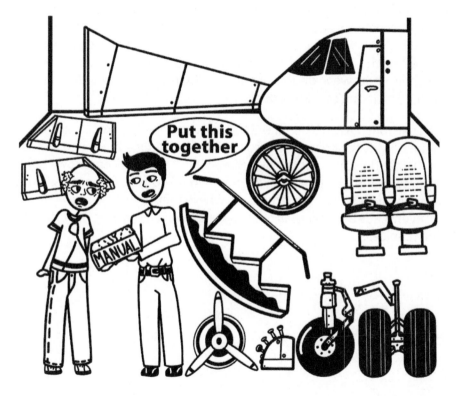

If you are planning to do a craft or a hobby, do not have all the pieces out on the table when the person with dementia enters. As a caregiver or an activity director, this can be difficult. Especially for those of us who like to plan ahead. When a person with dementia sees all that stuff out on the table, it can appear too overwhelming for them, and they will refuse or shut down. They go right back into the static. If they feel that it's too complicated, they're not even going to try. No way. Instead, only put out the first step or two, and as the activity progresses, introduce the next steps one at a time. Reassure them often that they are doing a great job.

People with dementia lose their executive-functioning skills. Executive functioning is the ability to perform steps in a particular order. It involves planning and sequencing. People with cognitive disabilities lose the ability to use this part of the brain. When someone begins to lose their executive functioning, they cannot sequence the correct order of steps or when seeing everything laid out in front of them, they become overwhelmed, thus shutting down and going into static mode. We can help overcome this very easily. An example of failing executive function would be when someone is no longer able to follow a recipe. Another would be when getting dressed, the cognitively impaired person may put their underwear on the outside of their pants rather than putting clothing on in the correct order.

Let's use lunch as an example. Going to a buffet-style restaurant would completely overwhelm the person, so would opening the fridge and asking, "What do you want to eat?" Simply limit the choices. Show them a can of tuna and a jar of peanut butter. "Would you like this or this?" They can point and choose. Depending on where they are in their disease, you will eventually be making all choices for them. "Here you go, eat this." No more choices.

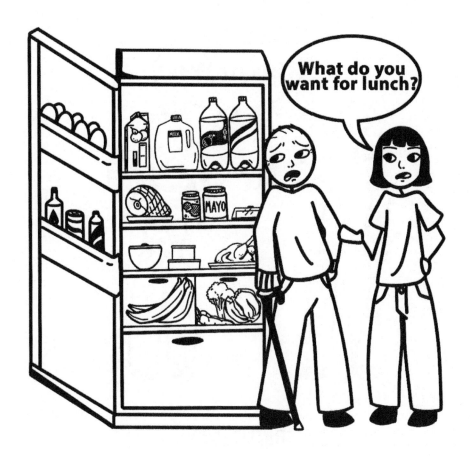

WRONG WAY

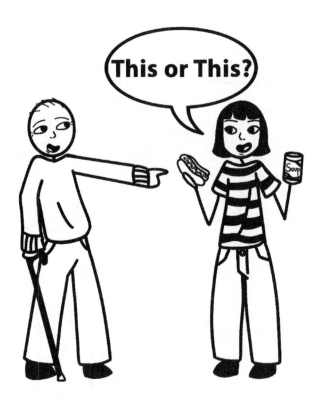

RIGHT WAY

Remember, activities make us who we are. So, how can we help them incorporate activities they once loved? This is so vital to their independence and self-confidence. Everyone must feel that they have a reason to exist. It is up to us, the cognitively intact, to help them maintain their self-esteem.

For a free download of activity ideas for early, middle, and late stages of dementia, visit our website at www.AnswersAboutAlz.org.

Suppose your person loved to golf. How can we find a way to simplify this activity or adapt it so they can still enjoy it? You could do some indoor putting. But instead of using a small cup, you could use a larger rectangular container, creating a much bigger opening to putt into. Stand closer to the target and putt the golf ball. In this way we can still have fun and feel connected to past activities. Success!

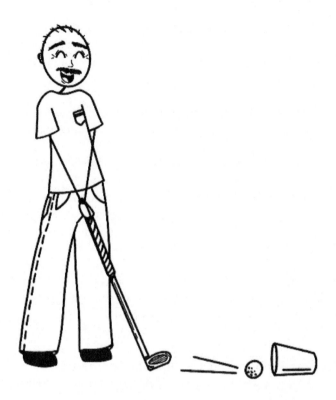

Process Over End Result!

If your loved one used to enjoy doing crossword puzzles but has lost interest, this is because they are no longer able to comprehend them or can no longer read. Go to the craft store or toy store and purchase some large letters. Ask them to spell their name with the letters. Maybe you could spell other simple words off that word, similar to a crossword puzzle. Be sure not to put too many letters out at a time. You could ask them, "What word could we spell off of that one?" After they say a word, then look for those letters, one at a time. If the activity becomes too difficult, put it away, and move on.

If someone loved to do a lot of traveling, you could look at photos from their past trips or look through travel books and magazines. Cut out pictures of interesting destinations. (Olivia, as your mom, this one will be good for me when I'm diagnosed. Just saying.)

Get creative on how to adapt activities to that person's past personal history. They'll thank you for your efforts. Actually, they probably won't. Caregiving is a thankless job-but I'll thank you on their behalf. THANK YOU!

Someone who loved to sew would enjoy manipulating and folding fabric swatches. Cut fabric or sort colorful spools of thread or bobbins.

A man who loved to tinker or fix things around the house would get joy out of a toolbox filled with nuts, bolts, nails, screws, washers, safety goggles, work gloves etc. Use your imagination. It can be very rewarding for you to put together meaningful activities for someone. There is no greater feeling than seeing their face light up when you give it to them. It's like Christmas morning!

A retired teacher would appreciate a blackboard, chalk, and an eraser. Play Tic Tac Toe. Ask her to teach you something. Give her self-esteem back to her. (We just did this for a retired teacher, and she absolutely loved it!)

If a task or activity becomes too difficult or creates frustration, end it immediately. Reassure them that it's okay, it's not a big deal, and move on to something else.

Exercise

How could you simplify the task of getting dressed for someone with Alzheimer's? Consider the steps, choices, and sequencing. Name three ideas. (Keep in mind the example of lunch.)

1. _____

2. _____

3. _____

What were some favorite activities that were important to the person you are caring for?

1. _____

2. _____

3. _____

4. _____

How can you incorporate/adapt some changes to that activity so they can still experience it?

_____

_____

_____

_____

Name three things you should do if the person is getting frustrated with an activity.

1. _____

2. _____

3. _____

List five new activity ideas that your loved one may enjoy.

1. _____

2. _____

3. _____

4. _____

5. _____

Reflection

We all need a purpose. Activities make us who we are and bring us joy. It's not about finishing the task. It does not have to be perfect. Lower expectations. Purpose vs perfection.

CHAPTER 5

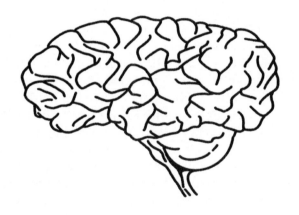

THESE DIVERSION TECHNIQUES CAN CHANGE YOUR LIFE!

Concept

In this case, Shiny Object Syndrome is a good thing! It's all about planning ahead. Having several strategies that are ready to go when we need a quick diversion can save your life and possibly your relationship.

Lesson

As humans, we will do almost anything to avoid boredom. Do you remember when you were a little kid? "Mom, I'm bored!" Begging Mom to help you get an activity started or give you an idea. Kids can't stand to be bored. They crave something to do. They'll go crazy just sitting around. What happens when a kid is not kept busy or occupied? They get into trouble, or they act out. They keep pestering you. Sound familiar? People with dementia want, need, and desire to be engaged. They want to be doing something. They need to be stimulated, but they can't get started. They can't come up with ideas on their own; they're stuck. They can't initiate. That's where we come in. We initiate.

What you don't know can hurt you. When it's been a long day, you're exhausted, and you need to distract your person with dementia, it's much easier if you have a plan of action!

Let me ask you this: Is it easier to start a conversation with a friend or a stranger? A friend, of course. That's because you know things about them. You know about their life, their family, their work, their habits. The more you know about the person you're caring for, the easier it will be to distract them. What are their favorite activities, favorite snacks, music, etc.? It's all about planning for the distraction. Personal history is your ammunition. So, start stockpiling the ammo! You're going to need it!

How about some more professional tips form Debra on distractions and activities? They're all yours by visiting our website at www. AnswersAboutAlz.org or our YouTube channel, Answers About Alzheimer's.

Get to Know Me

- What were/are their self-views?
- How do/did they see themselves?
- Where they an important figure, or one who stayed in the shadows?
- Where they socially active or a bit secluded?
- Where they a busy person?
- Couldn't sit still? Athletic?
- Always involved in a project?
- Were they quiet?
- A TV watcher?
- A book reader?

Every waking minute, our brains crave to be engaged in something. It doesn't matter what it is, as long as it's making us focus our attention to it. We seek entertainment. Our brains are designed to seek mental stimulation. Socialization, working, cooking, cleaning, watching TV, listening to music, taking care of personal hygiene, attending religious activities, and so on. The more we know about the person and their past experiences, the easier it will be to come up with effective distraction strategies. It is up to us, the cognitively intact, to make sure that they continue to feel and view themselves as an important individual with a purpose. What is life without a purpose? Meaningless.

How to Strategize

Stockpile your ammo. Your ammo is knowledge. Knowledge is power. Use it to your advantage. Start gathering.

- What are/were they most proud of?
- What was their life's work?
- Where did they live?
- Did they have pets growing up?
- What were Mom and Dad like?
- How was leisure time spent?
- Did they enjoy sports?
- Did they do volunteer work?
- Music preferences/styles

- Spiritual/religious history
- Favorite foods
- <u>Old</u> friends and family (not the grandchildren)
- Interests/hobbies
- Were they in the military?
- Who was important to them?
- What makes them laugh?

Effective diversions are your key to peace and happiness. When you discover what some of their favorite activities or shiny objects are, keep them handy for a quick diversion. (Also refer to "How to Keep 'em Busy in Ten Seconds or Less" chapter.)

- Look at <u>OLD</u> photo albums
- Sing a familiar song
- Watch a bird feeder
- Sort a big box of buttons
- Dance
- Give them something to hold
- Give them a job to "help you"
- A "rummage box" of things to sort/manipulate
- Fold towels (Over & over. They don't realize that you just asked them to help you. Mess them up and ask again. And again.)
- A jewelry box filled with costume jewelry (Me, me, me!)

For more incredible ideas visit us at <u>www.AnswersAboutAlz.org.</u>

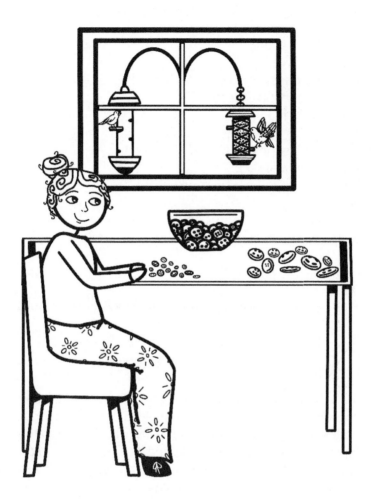

Ammunition Phrases for Distracting

If you take some time now to work on these, you will save valuable time and headaches down the road. Rehearse several of these to memory, so when you're "in the moment," you are well-prepared. Fill in the last of these sentences with a few options. Then, test them out and see which ones are the most effective and stick with the winners. Be sure your facial expressions and body language match the sentence. Be animated and excited to grab their attention! Their brain isn't getting your full energy level, so amplify the drama! Ramp it up!

- "Let's get your favorite…"
- "Hey, look at that cool…"
- "Here is your favorite…"
- "Show me your best…"
- "What is your most treasured…?"
- "Hey, I've got an idea…"
- "Let's go/do…".
- "I have a surprise for you. Come."
- "Let's find your dearest …"
- "You love _____, show me."
- "Come see…"
- "Look at this…"
- "What do you think…"
- "Can you help me with…"
- "Will you help me find…"

Do you want more? For the full list, go to www.AnswersAboutAlz.org.

Conversation Starters

You will have to decide to adapt these questions to present tense or past tense depending on the individual. Example: Tell me what your parents "did" OR tell me what your parents "do." (Never remind them that a loved one has passed away). So same as above, end these sentences with a few different ideas. Find which ones work well and keep using them over and over. Maintain eye contact, make sure they know you are listening, and that you are truly interested in what they are saying, even if you're really not. Fake it.

- "I'd love to hear about your favorite…"
- "Tell me about…"
- "When you were young…"
- "What were your family traditions…"
- "Have you done any traveling?"
- "Describe your holiday traditions."
- "What did/do your parents do for a living?"
- "What are some of your favorite past time activities/hobbies?"
- "What is your funniest story?"
- "Tell me about your family, where are they from?"

- "I love your collection of_____. Tell me about it."
- "What's the craziest thing you've ever done?"

OR

- Just start laughing hysterically.
- Start dancing.
- Sing a familiar song (*Happy Birthday, Row, Row, Row Your Boat, Tie a Yellow Ribbon, Amazing Grace*).
- Recite an old saying that would be familiar to them. (Nursery rhymes work well if they are in later stages of dementia.)

Play by Play

Grant keeps asking to go home. He is told over and over that we will be leaving soon, but he is in a repetitive state. His aide Jessica knows that Grant always had a bird feeder, and he can identify every bird in the area. Jessica asks Grant if he can help her identify the birds and grabs the bird book. She then asks for his "expert opinion" (making him feel important) about identifying some of the different species in the book. She asks what his favorite birds are and what they like to eat. They look out the window together and have a meaningful conversation about different species of birds. Jessica gives him power by telling him that she loves learning from him and that he is so knowledgeable and smart.

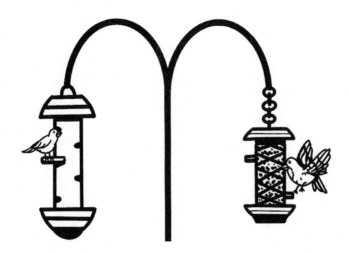

Rob keeps getting up from the dinner table and can't seem to sit still. This is very disruptive to the rest of the family, trying to enjoy hot meal. His daughter, Julie, has a couple of his favorite activities set aside for just this purpose. When Rob gets up this time, she's ready! She's got her ammunition! Rob's daughter grabs a container filled with different colored golf tees and ball markers. She dumps them on the table and asks him to "help her" by sorting them according to color. She knows her dad used to love to play golf and would be distracted by the golf tees and markers. If that didn't work, Julie has plan B ready. It's a sack filled with nuts and bolts and screws for him to sort and manipulate. Asking a person with dementia to "help you" by sorting items and getting the activity started is a great diversion technique. At the end, thank them for helping you. Tell them they are a lifesaver. "I don't know what I would have done without your help." "You're the best." When was the last time they felt important, valued, recognized? Recognize them for a job well-done!

Exercise

Using your knowledge from the "Keep 'em Busy" chapter and what you learned in this chapter, make recommendations for distracting the following people with dementia.

List five conversation starters

1. _____

2. _____

3. _____

4. _____

5. _____

List five Get to Know Me strategies you could use to distract.

1. _____

2. _____

3. _____

4. _____

5. _____

**Come up with three (different than above) ideas
to distract the following problems.**

Mary Ann is crying and feels afraid.

1. _____

2. _____

3. _____

**Dottie is looking for her mother who passed away
several years ago. (Three different.)**

1. _____

2. _____

3. _____

Harry wants to go to work. (Three different.)

1. _____

2. _____

3. _____

Reflection

People with Alzheimer's and dementia feel powerless. They do not have control over their thoughts and emotions, but they can be distracted. They need, want, and desire to be engaged in activities. Make their life easier by finding ways to interact with them and help them feel valued.

CHAPTER 6

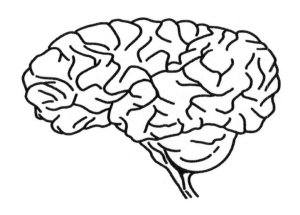

THE HORROR THEY SEE
THAT YOU DON'T

Concept

To most of us, interpreting our surroundings comes naturally. We don't even think about it. Your perception of your surroundings is completely different from those with dementia. Have you ever been in a haunted house? Where everything is distorted? Where everything is loud? You don't know what's coming at you. You don't know what to expect. Everything looks foreign or weird to you. You can't make sense of your surroundings. People with dementia are viewing their environment and saying, "Who are these people? I don't recognize them. Where am I? How do I get out of here? How do I escape? I'm petrified!"

Lucky for you, you can self-soothe, calm yourself, and eventually find your way out of the maze or a confusing, distorted setting. People with Alzheimer's or dementia cannot. They can't escape the confusion. They do not have the ability to self-soothe or self-calm. They are forced to be in this chaotic, frightening, confusing, environment 24/7! How scary! Just like a haunted house. No wonder they have behaviors!

In this chapter, we are going to learn that there are multiple things that can be done to alter their surroundings to make it more calming for people suffering from the disorienting effects of dementia.

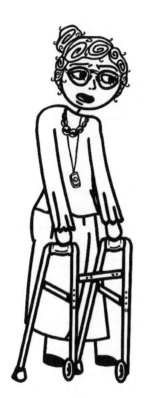

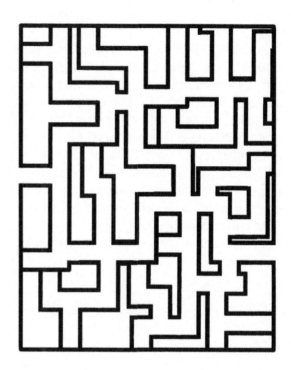

Even in familiar surroundings, the person with neuro- deficiencies will have difficulty navigating their environment.

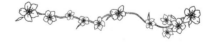

Lesson

When the cells of the temporal and parietal lobes of the brain are affected, the person will begin to have difficulties with visual-spatial and 3-D perception. This impairment alone can lead to behaviors and acting inappropriately. Their brain cannot interpret and process the information taken in by the eyes, ears, and other senses. Nor can the brain coordinate these efforts. Another function of the temporal and parietal lobes is the recognition of faces, objects, and judging distances. When this area of the brain is affected, we no longer recognize our loved ones, or understand how to use simple, everyday objects like silverware, toothbrushes, and walkers, and it throws off our balance, resulting in falls and confusion. The impact on vision and hearing is significantly increased above and beyond the normal aging process.

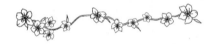

Sensory overstimulation increases confusion and reduces social interaction and affects self-esteem.

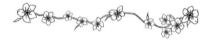

We must consider the following:

- Contrasting colors
- Monochromatic interiors
- Peripheral vision
- Depth perception
- Patterns
- Shadows

- Glare
- Environmental noise
- Temperature of the room (Refer to "Advice for Bathing from a Dementia Expert.")

Auditory Deficits

When we are in a room at a party and several conversations are occurring at once, we are able to "tune out" the background noise and focus on one conversation or listen to a presenter. We don't even think about it. If we lose focus for a moment, we are able to recognize it and return our attention back to that conversation. A person with Alzheimer's or dementia is unable to differentiate between the desired sounds and background noise.

Stop and take a moment to listen to all of the sounds you are hearing at any one time. Seriously, close your eyes and sit for about a minute and see how many different noises you are hearing at once. You will be surprised at how many you can identify. For example - a person talking, a TV, the hum of a dishwasher, a heater blowing, the birds and traffic outside, a dog barking. You probably didn't even notice all of those noises and you could choose to concentrate on one of those, filtering out the others. The person with dementia is hearing all of those noises at the same volume! The same volume! They cannot filter out the others. How can they possibly follow your request to get dressed or perform a simple task with all that noise going on in their head? When hearing deficits such as these present themselves, people withdraw from social activities. They avoid social interactions and become frustrated, isolated, agitated, confused, and have behaviors. Their world becomes increasingly smaller and smaller.

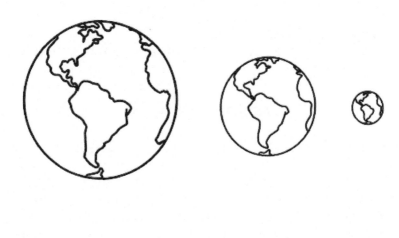

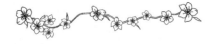

People with dementia have a decreased ability to decipher multiple, competing stimuli. Reducing the number of catalysts can significantly reduce frustration and confusion.

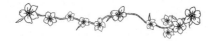

Reduce Audible Influences By

- Reduce the number of people in the room.
- Have only one person speak at a time.
- Turn off appliances or run them while they sleep.
- Turn off TVs.
- Use noise-canceling headphones.
- Reduce echoes using acoustic sound panels.

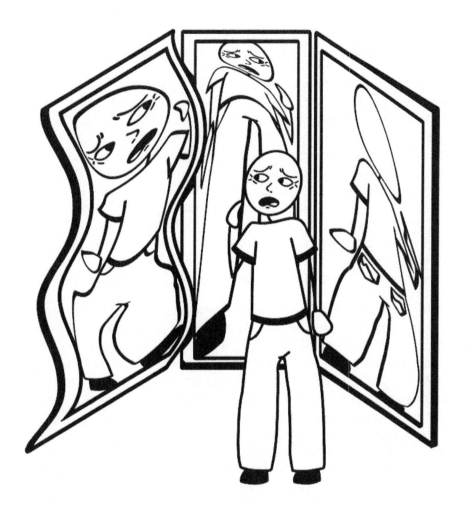

Visual Considerations

We observe the world around us as constantly moving and fluid. They see it as a motionless picture or photograph. Disjointed. Fragmented. Frame by frame. As we have learned so far, the Alzheimer's brain sees and interprets the environment in distorted ways. People with neu-ro-deficiencies cannot distinguish contrast, meaning that if a room has colors that are in the same shade range without a lot of contrast from light to dark, a person with dementia cannot see or interpret their sur-roundings. **(Visit our website at <u>www.AnswersAbourAlz.org</u> for more**

examples.) They have substantial problems with depth perception and peripheral vision that goes well beyond the normal aging process.

Consider being in a room where everything is white. (A little extreme, but you'll get the point.) The floor is white, the ceiling and walls are white, even the furniture is white. You cannot differentiate where the floor ends and the walls begin. It's very disorientating. It can through you off-balance. What if there is a dining room chair with a dark fabric seat sitting on a dark colored rug or dark hardwood flooring? They can't see where the seat is. It blends in with the floor. So, now let's say you have your mom in the bathroom where everything is the same color, and you tell her to sit on the toilet. She can't see it. She cannot see the toilet. How upset do you think someone would be if you're trying to tell them to sit on something that was invisible to them? They are not going to sit. They are afraid and anxious. It's just not going to work out very well.

As the disease progresses, it will become increasingly difficult for the person to see blues and greens. The color red is retained by the retina the longest. As I've stated before, it is imperative to use contrasting colors as much as possible. A bathroom can be particularly hard to navigate when the hues all blend together or are somewhat similar. A simple solution is to swap out the toilet seat for one that is red or black. This will make it much easier for them to see. If you do not have a walk-in shower, a quick and inexpensive solution is to put a stripe of bright yellow, orange, or red electrical tape across the edge of the tub or shower lip so they can navigate it better. Stairs can be very dangerous when considering the loss of depth perception. Again, we can edge each stair with a contrasting color tape, and use a different color to indicate the first and last step.

Lighting-Try to keep even lighting throughout the space. Dark spots and shadows can cause a feeling of discomfort and distress, causing confusion and increasing falls. Bright light throughout will help to provide a clearer picture of their surroundings. (See "The Ugly Truth About Sundowning" chapter.)

Just before I sent this book to the publisher, I went to meet a woman at a rehab for discharge. She is a retired social worker and she's traveled the world. Lynda has a diagnosis of Parkinson's and was experiencing dementia symptoms. I told her about the book and showed her a rough draft of the cover. When she looked at the picture, she tilted her head and said, "I see snakes." It's very interesting what people with dementia see and how they interpret their surroundings. Keep your eyes open and be curious about how they may be envisioning their surroundings.

Area rugs are not only a tripping hazard, but if they are a dark color, they can be perceived as a hole in the floor. The person who sees a hole in front of them will stop dead in their tracks. (This is a trick you can use for those exit seekers and wanderers!)

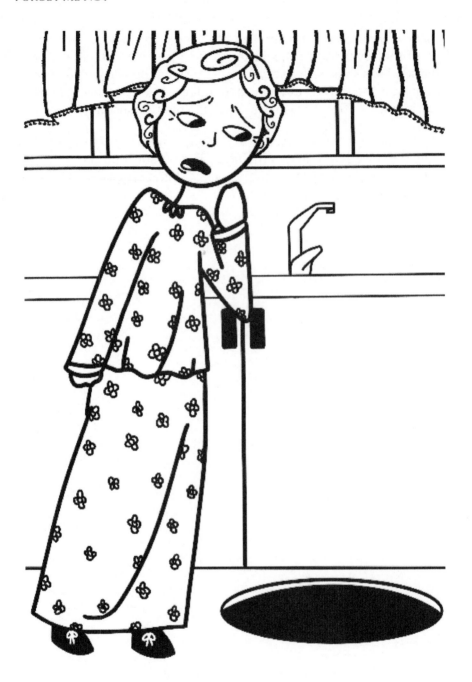

Bold patterns and prints can have different visual effects on people. These ornate patterns can play tricks on their mind. They can create confusion and disorientation. Zig-zags and stripes can appear as if they are moving. Florals or vine-like prints may appear to be snakes or other animals. Grid patterns, like a tile floor, can appear two-dimensional. Try walking on that! Shadows and glare can be very disturbing. Try to eliminate shiny or reflective surfaces. The reflective surfaces from china cabinets and mirrors can create confusion of the spatial relationship. Be cautious of pulsing shadows produced by ceiling fans. Reducing shadows is very important, especially if the person is suffering from sundowning. (Refer to "The Ugly Truth About Sundowning.") Poor lighting increases anxiety, behaviors, and increases the risk of falls.

Echoes- Large rooms that echo are very disturbing for those with cognitive disorders. Sound waves bounce back and forth off the walls and floors creating confusion. This phenomenon distorts how a person hears their own voice and the voices of others. Putting some canvas or cloth artwork on walls is one idea. You can easily add heavier window treatments, plants, or even install acoustic panels to absorb distorting sounds and vibrations.

I'm not saying you need to replace all your furniture or redecorate to accommodate the person with dementia, but there are an abundance of ways to inexpensively reduce visual and auditory stimuli, making it easier for them to navigate their environment.

Simple and Inexpensive Design Ideas to Reduce Negative Stimuli

- Drape solid color sheets over sofas and chairs that have large prints or patterns.
- Lay towels over the seat of dining chairs to contrast floor color.
- Put contrasting tape on tub edge.
- Use a contrasting toilet seat.
- Use contrasting tape on edge of stairs.
- Place contrasting tape on thresholds where different floor finishes come together.
- Use plates or placemats in a contrasting color from the table/foods

(red being best to contrast food.) (We can't see mashed potatoes on a white plate. Is that why they aren't eating? Can they see the food?)

- Close curtains to reduce shadows.
- Use contrasting floor-to-wall color or bright tape to outline the room.
- Reduce noise levels.
- Reduce echoes.

Visit **www.AnswersAboutAlz.org** for more examples.

Using Visual Cues

How old were you when you learned what a stop sign was? How old were you when you learned what a toilet was? The farther back that we learned something, the greater the chance we will remember it. If your loved one is not familiar with their surroundings anymore, you can try using pictures and signs to help them maintain independence. If there is a door that goes outside or leads into a basement, place a stop sign at their eye level or on the floor to deter them. Remember, people with dementia usually do not look up.

If they are experiencing confusion with toileting, one reason may be that they just don't know where the toilet is located, even if they have lived there for the past thirty years. Place a picture of a toilet on the door jamb entrance to the bathroom or on the floor to direct them. If they urinate on the picture on the floor, remove it. Lol. Sorry in advance if that happens. **Send your hate mail to Debra@AnswersAboutAlz.org.**

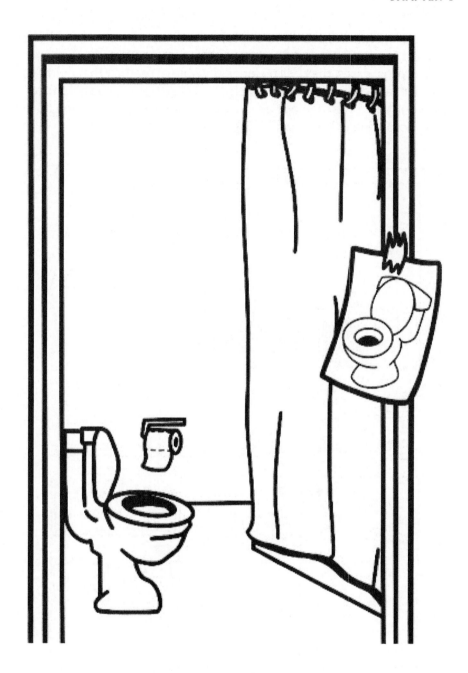

Pictures and notes can also be helpful on bedroom drawers and kitchen cabinets to locate items. At first, the written word may work, but as the disease progresses, they will no longer be able to read. At that point, you will change the written notes to pictures. These tips may be helpful for a while until the brain damage advances. Then we must adapt and adjust again, according to their ever-changing abilities.

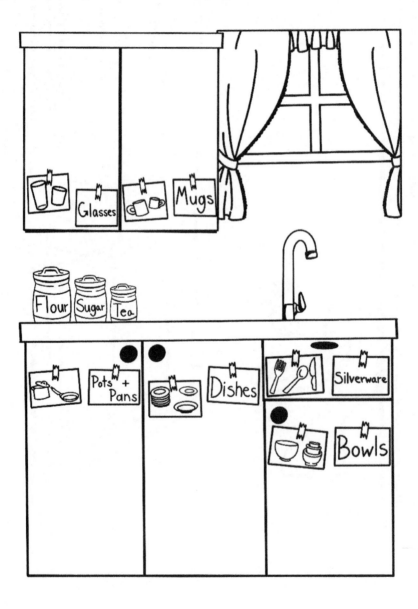

Play by Play

I went to visit Roderick and Teresa a few years ago. They lived in an old house in the heart of the city. Roderick was the caregiver for his wife who had Alzheimer's. He was an engineer, and she had raised the family. Their living room was made up primarily of dark, antique furniture, dark shag carpeting, and not a lot of natural light. They spent the majority of their time in the living room, and each of them had a favorite reclining chair. Roderick's was burgundy and Teresa's was green. I'm sure most of us have our special spot that we always sit in. Teresa was declining and her daughter came for a visit from California. While I was talking with the family, Teresa got up from the dining room table and was not sure where to go. The daughter repeatedly told Mom, "Go sit in your green chair. Go sit in your green chair, Mom." I explained to her that her mom could no longer decipher blues and greens, and at this point she might not even recognize what the word "color" meant. It would be easier for her to understand if she just referred to it as "your chair." With her advanced cognitive decline, we should be shortening these sentences. "Go sit" or "This way" and lead her to her chair.

Olivia led her client Bonnie into the bathroom to take a shower. As Olivia started to undress Bonnie, she was clearly getting confused and disoriented. Olivia was now trying with all her might to encourage Bonnie to step over the edge of tub and get into the shower. Bonnie was paralyzed and she was shaking. She was clearly confused and afraid. Bonnie was feeling very overwhelmed. She couldn't make sense of her environment. It was too loud, and she couldn't see the edge of the tub, but Olivia kept repeatedly instructing her on what to do. Everything in the bathroom was the same color. Bonnie no longer had depth perception and couldn't see the tub against the floor. She was terrified that she would fall down and drown. People with dementia have a tremendous fear of drowning.

Instead, try this- Olivia went into the bathroom before bringing Bonnie in and prepared for a shower. She made sure the room was warm. Very warm. Olivia placed a wide stripe of bright red tape across the edge of the tub so Bonnie could see it. She also gathered all of the supplies she would need ahead of time. Olivia decided to leave the fan off until Bonnie was finished and out of the bathroom. She handed her a washcloth to hold for comfort. (Also refer to "Advice for Bathing from a Dementia Bathing Expert" chapter.)

Exercise

How can you make the bathroom environmentally friendly and easier to navigate for the person with dementia?

_____

_____

_____

What are some steps you could take to reduce the noise levels in the home or community?

_____

_____

_____

When considering how the person with dementia sees their surroundings, what other things can you look for that may be disturbing to them?

_____

_____

_____

Suzie moved her mother into her home with her. It is a big, beautiful house with an open floor plan. What environmental factors should Suzie be considering?

_____

_____

_____

How can I reduce noise levels in the environment?

_____

_____

_____

Reflection

It's like living in a haunted house. Everything is distorted. They can't make sense of their surroundings. They cannot escape the confusion. People with dementia are forced to live in a haunted house 24/7. Look for ways to add contrast to the environment.

CHAPTER 7

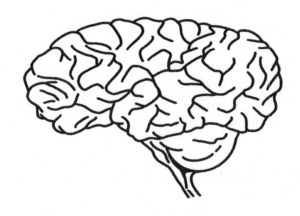

THE UGLY TRUTH ABOUT
SUNDOWNING

Concept

Sundowning or Sundown Syndrome. What the heck is that? Sundowning seems like a big mystery and sounds complicated. The truth is, it's not!

Lesson

It's crazy time! Here comes the split personality. Everyday around this time, she loses it. Sundowning is a group of symptoms and behaviors that a person with dementia suffers later in the afternoon and evening and can continue on through the night. It typically begins as the sun goes down. For approximately 25 percent of people with Alzheimer's, this syndrome will develop during the middle to late stages of dementia. Researchers do not know the exact cause, but some speculate that it has something to do with the internal clock or circadian rhythms. The person's dementia symptoms are much more intense than usual if they are sundowning.

What Causes Sundowning?

Many believe it is simply exhaustion at the end of the day, and still others hypothesize it is due to changes in lighting, which in turn causes disorientation and peaks agitation. Increased shadows can disorient and confuse a person with dementia. They cannot orientate to their surroundings. Whatever the reason, there are things we can do to significantly reduce these behaviors. (Refer to "The Horror They See That You Don't" chapter, especially shadows and glare.)

Sundowning Symptoms

Do you observe a significant contrast in behaviors from morning/daytime compared to afternoon/evening hours?

Anxiety	Delusions
Heightened confusion	Hallucinations
Fatigue	Screaming/yelling
Anger	Exit seeking
Wandering	Resistance
Pacing	Disorientation
Agitation	Suspicions

The burden of sundowning can be monumentally challenging for family members, caregivers, and staff. The most important thing to remember is, this too shall pass. People who are suffering from dementia require more sleep. Limiting naps to one hour or less will help to keep the circadian rhythm on the right track. Included in the symptoms of sundowning, people can have difficulty differentiating dreams from reality. (Refer to "Advice for Behaviors You'd be Crazy Not to Take" chapter.)

Shadows cast by the sun going down are confusing and disorientating to the person with dementia, even frightening. Keep the blinds closed to reduce shadows and turn on lights. Referring to what we have learned about the environment, during these heightened episodes, keep the environment quiet. Reduce stimulation and limit background noise. (Refer to "The Horror They See That You Don't.") If the person is pacing, let them be. They may just need to move. The sundowning person may follow you around closely and repeat the same question over and over. It's not about the question, it's about the concern behind the question. They are afraid. They feel like they should be doing something, but they cannot initiate a task. They just do not know what to do with themselves. Try to engage them in an activity (Refer to "How to Keep 'em Busy in Ten Seconds or Less") or ask them if they will "help you" with something important. Actually, tell them it's an important assignment. People with dementia like to help others. It makes them feel important.

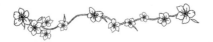

IF THEY ARE SAFE, LET THEM PACE!

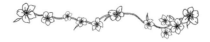

If the person has a favorite activity, try redirecting to that activity. Music may help. Studies show that sundowning symptoms of agitation, aggression, and depression improved with thirty minutes of music therapy three times a week. Music therapy can mean simply playing their favorite music, not necessarily a formal music program. Reassure them using your gentle touch and soft calming voice. Let them know everything is okay and you are there to support them. If the person is angry, let them know you understand and that you will do your best to make it better. ("Validate and Captivate" chapter.) A person with dementia wants to be heard and understood. This is when you are going to use your safe words and stay clear of trigger words. ("How to Talk So They'll Listen" chapter.) Dealing with hallucinations can be particularly challenging. It is vital that you do not tell them they are hallucinating. This is also not something you should disagree with or argue about. Remember, you cannot argue with a person with dementia. If the hallucinations are frightening or upsetting to them and all your attempts to divert and redirect fail, it may be time to have the neurologist intervene and prescribe an anti-psychotic drug. Again, be reassuring. Hallucinations are covered in depth in the "Advice for Behaviors You'd be Crazy Not to Take."

Rule Out

Need to toilet	Uncomfortable clothing
They are looking for something	Pain
They are looking for someone	Hunger

Thirsty

Hot

Cold

UTI

Sundowning Solutions

Close the blinds

Turn on lights

Avoid caffeine/alcohol

Play favorite music

Reduce noise

Reduce stimuli

Redirect to an activity

More exercise during the day if awake at night

Melatonin to help sleep at bedtime

More sunlight during daylight hours

Easier tasks

Reassure them

Vitamin D

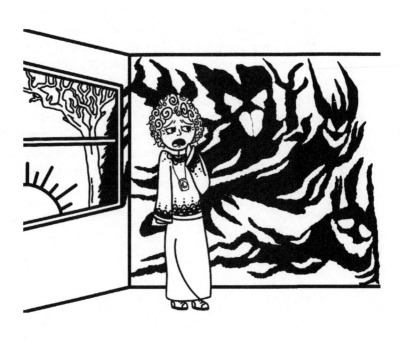

When a person is experiencing sundowning, they have trouble making sense of their environment. Shadows and glare can be especially disturbing, causing confusion. These disturbances can manifest into behaviors of anxiety, aggression, irritability, fear, a feeling of loss of control, and elopement.

Play by Play

You Can Help!

Dorothy is sundowning. As late afternoon approaches, Dorothy's behavior changes. It's like she's a different person. Her dementia symptoms go through the roof, and she becomes unmanageable. She paces, exit seeks, and gets angry easily. She's so nervous and jittery. Dorothy's caregiver has a new plan of action. Knowing that these symptoms are coming, the caregiver can plan and prepare. Before lunch, they go for a walk to stretch and get some exercise and sunshine. It is believed that getting ten minutes of sunshine per day (preferably in the morning) can resynchronize your circadian rhythm or the sleep-wake cycle. Even sitting by a window can be beneficial. Before the sun starts setting, the caregiver closes all the blinds and curtains and turns on all the lights to minimize shadows. We know that Dorothy enjoys manipulating fabric and used to be a seamstress. We have a sewing box filled with different fabrics and ribbons to distract her into an activity that she enjoys. We also know that she loves caramel candies and have a few of those on hand. She seems to respond better when we have a big smile and reassure her that we are feeling the same way she is feeling and that we are right by her side. By reassuring Dorothy and having several activities planned, closing the blinds, and creating a less stimulating environment around her, we have greatly reduced Dorothy's anxiety and sundowning symptoms. (Refer to "Validate and Captivate.")

Exercise

Millie is on the move. She will not sit still. It is 5:30 p.m. I just got home from work. I am exhausted and need to make dinner for the family. Millie is driving me crazy. Walking back and forth, back and forth. She just won't stop following me around. She's like my shadow!

What three things can we do for Millie?

1. _____

2. _____

3. _____

Every evening, my husband, Bud, gets really agitated and incredibly angry. Bud acts out by yelling and swearing. Sometimes he gets so angry, he slams his fists on the table.

How can you help Bud?

_____

_____

_____

If I have someone who is suffering from sundowning, I can try to rule out the following:

_____

_____

_____

Some things I can do to help someone with sundowning symptoms are:

_____

_____

_____

My patient/family member is pacing. I should...

_____

_____

_____

Reflection

People with dementia become tired and agitated later in the day. Close the blinds and turn on the lights to reduce shadows that can be distracting and disturbing. Reduce activities, redirect, and reassure them. Stay calm, it won't last forever.

CHAPTER 8

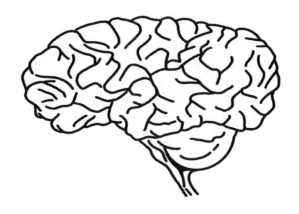

ADVICE FOR BATHING
FROM A DEMENTIA EXPERT

Concept

I know you mean well. But when you understand what that resistant person is feeling, and what their brain is perceiving in the shower, you will realize that you are torturing them. You must stop pushing this issue. Forcing a person with dementia to take a shower is ABUSE! JUST STOP! In most cases, when I explain to a family member what's really happening in their brain, they start crying. It's not your fault, you didn't know.

Lesson

We've all been there. The bathing blues. What we wouldn't give to make the bathing experience easier! As this disease progresses, the person with dementia no longer understands the purpose of bathing or personal hygiene. After age sixty-five, we begin to significantly lose our sense of smell, so they don't realize that they have an odor problem.

Let's face it, bathrooms are cold, hard, and just plain scary for people with dementia. And on top of all that, we expect them to take off their clothes. Getting naked in front of another person isn't easy unless your past history was regularly visiting a nude beach. (I went once, it was awesome!) Reflecting on "The Horror They See That You Don't" chapter, you will recall that many bathrooms are monochromatic. Everything is the same color or hues. There isn't enough contrast. A person with dementia cannot see a white tub on a white floor against a white wall. They cannot see the edge of the tub to step over it. No matter how many times you tell them, you can't make them see something that they don't see. People with cognitive challenges have multiple vision deficiencies way above and beyond the normal aging process. A simple and inexpensive trick is to put a strip of sharply contrasting tape across the edge of the tub so they can see it. Preferably red, as red is retained the longest by the retina. If you can make the bathroom an inviting space, rather than a scary, cold, loud space, it will greatly increase your chances of success. And I am going to teach you exactly how to do it! You're welcome!

Why won't they?

- The room is too cold
- Fear of falling
- Fear of drowning
- Embarrassment
- Pain
- Confusing environment
- Too loud
- Task is too complicated
- Purpose of bathing is forgotten
- Sex of the helper

If you are able, find out what the person's past bathing habits and preferences were. Did they prefer a shower or a bath? What time of day did they like to shower? Was it first thing in the morning or immediately after the evening news? Can you see how this information can help you? Consider this, many people with dementia perform tasks better earlier in the day before they get tired out.

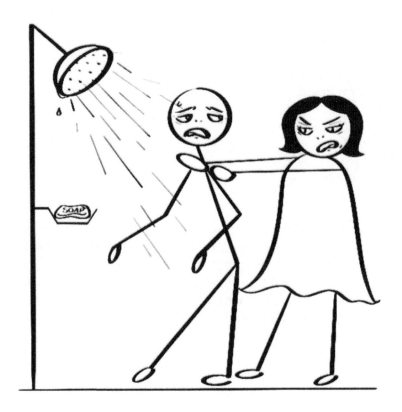

WRONG WAY

How many times a week should they bathe?

Seniors don't sweat nearly as much, so unless they are having other issues such as incontinence or don't use toilet paper effectively, once or twice a week should be fine. Speaking of not using toilet paper efficiently, a bidet is a WONDERFUL solution for both the caregiver and your loved one. A bidet can be installed right on your existing toilet. It will gently clean their private areas with a warm water spray and then dry them off! Oh hell yeah!

Try creating an inviting environment. Bathrooms tend to be an extremely personal space. It is where we go for privacy. It's uncomfortable to be in there with other people. Bathrooms are loud and echoey. They are hard, cold, and uncomforting spaces. Try to create a more inviting, cozy space that they would enjoy. Use some flameless candles, soft music, or fancy soaps. Remember your safe words from the communication chapter. Spa day, wash up, freshen up. Perhaps, "Let's have a girl's spa day and we can do your hair and nails. Yay! Won't that be fun?" "I have your favorite soap." Don't forget your body language. If you have your hands on your hips and say, "Time for a shower," they're going to give you a fight. If your attempts are just not going to work out today, retreat, and try again later or even tomorrow. Remember to be flexible. Lower expectations. Don't argue with a person with dementia. You will only get MORE resistance.

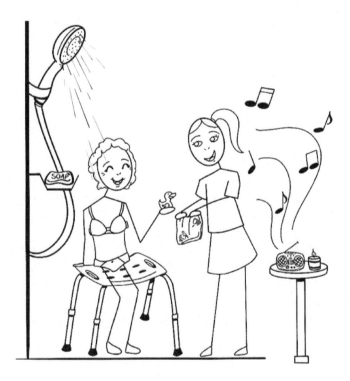

RIGHT WAY

Visit my YouTube channel, Answers About Alzheimer's for more bathing and toileting tips.

Play by Play

Shower Comfort Tips

- Pad the shower chair with a thick, fluffy, triple-folded towel.
- Give them something to hold for a sense of security (washcloth, shampoo bottle, tell them it's their job to hold it), a rubber duck. (Tell them it's a good luck duck.)
- Warm the bathroom.
- Play music or sing songs (not **your** favorite music, **their** favorite music.)
- Fancy soaps/aromatherapy (Tell them it's fancy soap, let them smell it.)
- Monitor the water temperature.
- Cover private areas with a towel.
- Keep undergarments on until washing that part of the body.
- Have them do as much as possible for themselves (especially private parts).
- Have them wash their own face. (It's terrifying to have someone come towards your face. Go ahead, try putting your hand in someone's face and see what happens.)
- Invest in a towel warmer.
- I hope I don't have to say grab bars! And never the suction-cup style!

NEVER POUR WATER OVER SOMEONE'S FACE!

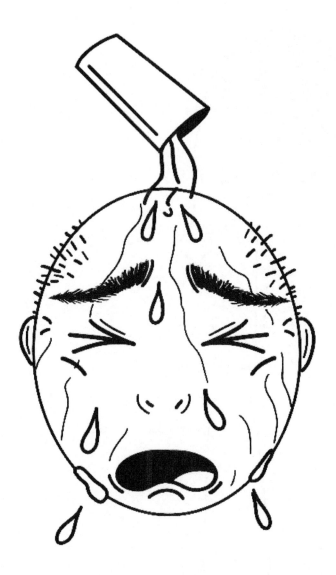

People with dementia are ultra-sensitive to touch due to the damage to the braincells. Be very gentle. Use a soft touch when washing delicate skin, and pat dry, do not rub.

To Bathe or Not to Bathe!
Not happening! No way!

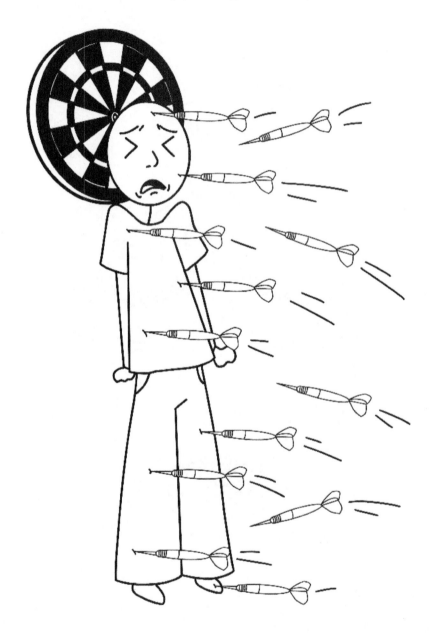

Why Do They Refuse?

The Alternative

You're welcome! Again! In the mid-to-later stages of Alzheimer's and dementia, a shower will become a painful experience. The beads of water actually feel like needles and pin pricks due to the sensory perception from damage to the brain. It hurts. A lot! Would you like a spray of needles hitting you all over your naked body? Would you like to feel like a dart board? If your person is resistant to taking a shower, there are alternatives that are just as good as a full shower experience. Your loved one will not suffer or get sick if they cease showering forever. This is YOUR perception! Your bias. You can purchase no-rinse bathing cloths or towels. These bathing towels are enriched with aloe and are alcohol-free. Exposing and washing one area at a time with the warm towels is a luxurious experience. Shampoo caps are available to wash hair with no water needed. Simply heat in the microwave and put the warm cap on the head and gently massage, remove, and style as usual. Most people love this option. Many people with dementia feel like they are getting a comforting, warm massage and actually enjoy the experience! Imagine that! They actually like it! Shampoo caps and disposable bathing towels are the perfect solution to the bathing blues.

Refer to the chapter, "Advice for Behaviors You'd Be Crazy Not to Take," and our website at www.AnswersAboutAlz.org for additional information and training concerning inappropriate behaviors and sexual expression during bathing and other activities.

Exercise

My person's past bathing habits and preferences are/were?

_____

_____

_____

Name three reasons why someone is reluctant to get in the shower.

1. _____

2. _____

3. _____

I can make the bathing experience easier by doing these five things.

1. _____

2. _____

3. _____

4. _____

5. _____

I will never _____ over someone's face.

Reflection

Bathing is painful for me. It hurts me. I am scared. I am cold. I am embarrassed. I have trouble navigating a monochromatic environment. Give me something to hold in the shower for comfort. Be patient with me, I don't understand. It's okay if I don't shower ever again. There are alternatives.

CHAPTER 9

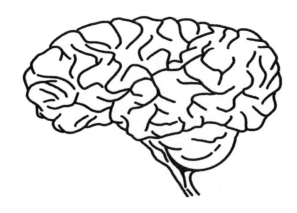

THE UNTOLD DANGERS
OF DEMENTIA

Concept

Safety Concerns- It's not a matter of **"IF,"** it's a matter of **"WHEN."**

Common dangers include:

- Fire
- Overdose
- Firearms
- Poisoning
- Wandering/Exit seeking
- Drowning
- Motor vehicle accidents

Lesson

Our brains are made up of billions of neurons. These neurons are responsible for getting information, processing information, and sending out information. Neurons communicate with each other through electrical charges and are interconnected to approximately ten thousand other neurons. When these neurons die, it creates gaps, and the information can no longer cross over to be received, processed, or stored.

Think of the neurons in the brain as if they were a huge map. A map of many, many roads and bridges. You're driving down the road, and all of a sudden, there is a roadblock. You stop suddenly and have nowhere to go. You just stop. A person with dementia can be performing a task, and suddenly the bridge is gone. Just like that! Their brain has nowhere to go. They very simply forget what they are doing. They just stop. This is when a person with dementia is in danger of hurting themselves or putting others at risk. There is no way to predict when this will happen, so we must prepare for it ahead of time.

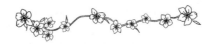

It's not a matter of "IF,"
It's a matter of "WHEN."

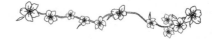

I never like to compare an adult with dementia to a child; however, when it comes to safety, that is the most accurate comparison. Those with Alzheimer's or other related dementias, no longer understand consequences for actions. They do not process outcomes for their choices. Actions are irreversible. They no longer comprehend what danger is.

Safety Tips

Exit Seeking and Wandering

When elopement and exit seeking threatens safety, you don't have time to figure things out. The time is now! Bed and chair alarms can be life-savers. Doors must also be locked and alarmed. You can disguise exit doors to look like a continuation of the wall, put a poster of a landscape to look like a window, or put a window treatment on the door. Place a large plant in front of an exit door. You can also put stop signs on exits to deter a person with dementia. Remove trigger items such as purses, coats, and shoes. Hang bells on doorknobs in the bedroom to alert a sleeping spouse. People with dementia tend not to look up. Slide bolt locks can be easily installed up high. Exit seeking and wandering are covered in-depth in the "Advice for Behavior You'd be Crazy Not to Take," and "The Horror They See That You Don't" chapters.

Poison Control

Lock up all cleaning supplies and potential poisons. Don't forget the garage and basement.

Medications

All medications should be locked up and a responsible person should give meds as needed.

Fire Safety

Install a shut-off valve for a gas stove, or a circuit breaker for electric stoves. Remove knobs from stoves. Do not use toaster ovens. Make sure you have working fire extinguishers, smoke detectors, and carbon monoxide detectors. Discard all matches and lighters.

Firearms

Remove all firearms, weapons, and ammunition from the home.

Car keys

Hide car keys or dismantle the car engine.

PERS or GPS

Invest in a good Personal Emergency Response System (PERS) or GPS locator for the person with dementia to wear.

Shoe Tracking Devices

Shoe inserts that will track wandering.

Tools and Equipment

Lock up any potentially dangerous tools, ladders, power tools, and farm equipment.

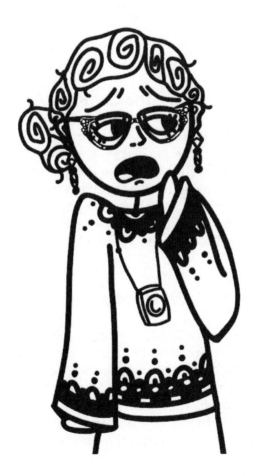

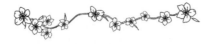

Remember a person with cognitive disabilities will not be able to dial 911, recall their address, or get out safely.

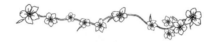

How To Take the Car Keys Away

Telling a parent that they need to stop driving is a conversation most of us put off as long as possible. No matter when these conversations take place, it's usually not pretty. Try to see things from their perspective. This is a debilitating blow to their independence. You must choose your words carefully. Be gentle and show concern for safety. It's all about safety, not, "You can't, you shouldn't." (Remember your safe words from the "How to Talk, So They'll Listen" chapter.)

What can I do?

- Have a frank but calm discussion. Several if possible. Ask Mom or Dad for their input on solutions and brainstorm together.
- Talk to Mom or Dad's doctor. (Ask the doctor to recommend a driving evaluation.) Attempt to get Mom and Dad to commit to doing whatever the driving evaluation results recommend.
- In extreme circumstances, dismantle the car engine so it will no longer run. For example, disconnect the battery or remove the distributor cap.
- Hide the vehicle or take away the car keys.
- Contact the DMV to report unsafe driving.

The key is to find Mom and Dad several alternative means of transportation before taking the car away. It is much harder to argue a point when you already have a solution to the problem in place. Examples may be friends, family, Uber, or a local senior transportation service. Ask a family member to commit to taking Mom shopping once a week. Have a friend from church volunteer to pick Mom up every Sunday for church services. Plan to have a friend from the bridge club come to carpool with Mom to play bridge every Wednesday evening. Give Mom the name and phone number for a local transportation company and tell her she can call at any time and go anywhere she wants. Mom needs to be reassured that she will not miss out on any events or functions by giving up driving. Most importantly, you must come through with the promises you make.

Explain that you are concerned for their safety, and you want them around for years to come. Your parent may feel they will have fewer trips outside the home. They worry that they will become isolated, have increased dependency on others, fewer social outings, and they fear becoming a burden to family and friends. These are valid concerns. Discuss these as openly as possible.

What can I say?

Do NOT say, "You need to stop driving," or "You shouldn't be driving anymore." Instead, talk about safety. "I worry about you," or "It would be awful if you were in an accident and hurt yourself or someone else." Calmly bring up any medical conditions, medications for pain that may cause dizziness, vision problems, and hearing loss. Most importantly, tell them you love them. This is a big blow to their freedom and independence. The transition can be difficult, and it can take some time to get used to. Speak from the heart. Be patient and diligent; it will get better with time.

As we have learned in previous chapters, you cannot reason with someone with dementia, so unless these conversations are happening at the very beginning of their journey, you may have to jump in and take matters into your own hands. Unfortunately, there comes a day when you, as the cognitively intact, must make safety decisions for your loved one. Remember, eventually there will be no more choices. It's hard to play the bad guy, but think about what could and will happen. You don't want to be regretting that for the rest of your life. Trust me, been there, done that!

To hear Debra's heartbreaking story of Alzheimer's, elder abuse, and murder, visit www.AnswersAboutAlz.org.

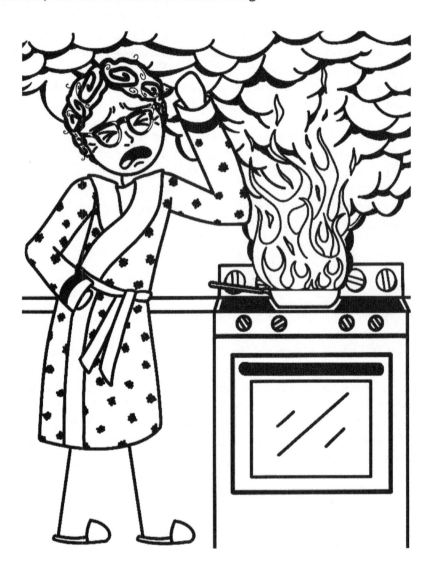

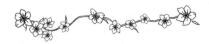

When it is questionable whether or not a person would be able to get out of the home independently under the circumstance of an emergency, it's time for 24-hour supervision.

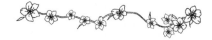

Play by Play

True Story

There was a man living alone whose wife had recently passed away. He had undiagnosed dementia. The family, consisting of five children, all had a different idea on how much care and supervision Dad needed. They went back and forth between 24-hour care and several hours per day shared with his high school-aged grandchildren who lived across the street. One day, when it was time for the caregiver to leave, the family said they were on their way over and sent the aide home. After the caregiver left, she realized that she had left some important papers behind. She was gone perhaps all of five minutes. She pulled back into the driveway, and when she got out of her car, she heard wails of terror coming from the garage. She ran towards the horrific cries and found her client completely engulfed in flames. A blowtorch was lying on the concrete floor beside him. She managed to get him into the shower and called 911. Tragically, he had severe burns covering most of his body, and his pants had melted to his legs. He passed away after several painful days in the hospital.

Fact

It was the first day that the caregiver was working for the sweet elderly couple. She was told the wife had Alzheimer's. The caregiver was making lunch for the couple when the wife approached her with a bottle of Mr. Clean and asked her if she would like some juice! When the caregiver brought this to the attention of the husband, he replied, "Yeah, she does stuff like that sometimes." At the same home, the caregiver discovered that the very thin dog was being fed packaging Styrofoam peanuts instead of dog food. Fluffy was promptly rehomed to a family member.

Really Happened

Betty was a highly active senior. Her favorite activity was swimming. She went to the local YMCA at least three times a week to swim laps. Betty could no longer drive because she would forget where she was going and got lost easily. Her son had been advised that swimming might not be a safe activity for his mother any longer, but he insisted that it was an important part of her life and good for her to get exercise. The following Monday, Betty went to the YMCA, escorted by her friend. She got into the pool and began to swim. Halfway across the pool, she forgot what she was doing. She just stopped swimming! She sank to the bottom like a stone. It took three visits and three lifeguard rescues before the YMCA told her she could no longer return.

Legit

An elderly couple was vacationing at their cottage in the Thousand Islands. She had spent her life's work in service helping others as a social worker at the hospital. Marguerite was French and loved to cook. This particular evening, however, she was cooking at the stove, forgot what she was doing, and she just walked away, leaving the stove unattended. It wasn't long before a fire broke out. Thankfully, her husband Mike was close by. He was able to quickly extinguish the fire before it got out of control. Marguerite was no longer allowed to cook.

Seriously

Once upon a time there was a lovely couple named Art and Doris who lived in the city. They had lived in this house for over forty-five years. One cold, frosty night in January, Doris decided she wanted to go home. (She was looking for the home she grew up in.) She left the house with no shoes or coat, bound and determined to go home. After several failed attempts to convince her to come back, the last resort was to call 911 and initiate a mental hygiene arrest. This was a very traumatic event for both Doris and her husband. Shortly after that incident, it was decided that Doris had to be moved to a memory care unit for her safety.

No Lie

A gentleman named James woke up in the middle of the night and was confused. His surroundings looked unfamiliar, and he did not know where he was. In his state of confusion, he made it outside without waking his sleeping wife. Several hours later, his wife awoke to realize that James was not in the bed next to her. After frantically searching the house, she called 911 and her daughter. The police came quickly, and it didn't take the authorities long to find him. He had taken a left-hand turn at the end of the driveway and walked right over the cliff. He suffered several broken bones and a concussion but survived his injuries. He spent several weeks in the hospital and a month in rehab.

For Real

Myron, Myron, Myron! Oh, what are we going to do about Myron? Myron loved his candles. They were everywhere. He had a habit of burning small votive candles on paper plates. Every day that we came to visit, the caregiver would find burnt matches on the paper plates with the melted remains of the candles. After several attempts to remove all the matches from his home, day after day, we continued to find more burnt matches everywhere, on every surface in the house. So, one day we went to the Christmas Tree Shop and bought a wide assortment of flameless candles, brought them to Myron, and showed him the newest, latest, and greatest invention of all time! We convinced him to give up his old boring candles and replace them with the new, cool flameless candles. It worked!

No Joke

Helen was living in a memory care unit. Her only companion was her cat, Bubblez. Helen loved her cat. The community's policy was that you were allowed have a pet as long as you were able to take care of it. Helen's family knew how much Bubblez meant to her, so when she could no longer feed the cat, they hired an outside agency to help out. Shortly after the aides started coming to attend to the cat's needs, they discovered that Helen was eating the clumps in the litter box. It was time to find a new home for the beloved cat. A mechanical cat was promptly introduced to Helen. Thankfully, at this later stage of her disease process, she didn't even know the difference.

Honestly True

At an assisted living community on a frigid February night, an elderly man walked out of the building unnoticed by staff. The next day after breakfast, he was reported missing. The search lasted a couple of days. The man's body was finally found in the frozen pond on the grounds of the community, not far from the main entrance.

Walkers and Canes

What I'm about to tell you, you may find hard to believe. I struggled with this concept myself at first.

Assistive-walking devices are designed for safety. They were developed to help maintain balance and stability while walking. However, these aids must be used in the way in which they were intended, or they can become a tripping hazard. In order to have a safe, successful outcome, a person needs to be able to demonstrate reliable, consistent, and proper use of the equipment. Do you have to remind your loved one every single time they get up to use their walker? Over and over, they never remember to use it? You're so worried about a fall. You can't be there 24/7. What are you to do? You're not alone.

Insisting that Mom or Dad use an assistive-walking device, may actually be doing them more harm than good, but I'll explain that a little later.

Alzheimer's not only affects memory, thinking, and language, but it also impairs movements and bodily functions. People who have cognitive disabilities are not able to rely on short-term memory. They are not capable of learning new concepts or equipment. They lack the capacity to take a newly learned skill and store it into their long-term memory to retrieve it later. So, if we introduce new equipment, they will either forget that they need to use it, or they won't remember how to use it properly. The exception to this is if the walker or cane was introduced prior to the onset of symptoms.

People with dementia do not understand the reasoning behind using a device. They no longer understand consequences for actions. Therefore, they don't recognize a safety issue. You cannot make them understand, and you cannot make them remember to use the walker no matter how hard you try. I know you mean well, and you're doing your best, but this is not a battle you will win. They just don't get it. They can't help it. It's the loss of brain cells.

Multi-tasking with cognitive decline is impossible for the compromised person. Walking with or without an assistive device is a multi-tasking skill. Walking and navigating the environment requires a tremendous amount of brain bandwidth. Coordinating movement and balance takes significant cognitive power.

Think about everything that goes into the physical task of walking. We must plan our route. We need to consider our destination and have a reason for going to that destination. We must use our motor skills, our muscular and skeletal systems, and we need to use balance along with our visual and auditory senses. For us to walk, all of these systems must come together. Coordination of all of these actions requires executive functioning. A person with Alzheimer's or dementia no longer has executive functioning or sequencing skills. This loss happens early in the progression of Alzheimer's disease. It takes an incredible amount of effort to walk with a purpose, a destination, and coordinate a walker or cane.

Maneuvering a walker for a person with dementia is a complex motor skill activity. It's the equivalent of texting and driving. We all know that's a disaster waiting to happen. How many things can you do at any one time before causing an accident?

Putting our cognitive demands into using a walking device leads to unstable gait, accelerates task complexity, and increases the demand on our brain, which raises the risk of falls.

For people with dementia, the fact is, they are three times more likely to fall when using a walker versus not using anything at all.

In a healthy adult, it was found that it took only slightly more cognitive work to manipulate a walker, but the workload increased by approximately 40 percent for people with dementia.

In conclusion, studies show that mobility aids and walkers should be reconsidered for the person who has Alzheimer's or other dementias.

(If the final decision is still to introduce a walker to the person with dementia, I recommend prepping it to be attractive to them. Personalize the equipment as much as possible. First, put their first name, big and bold, facing the inside where the person will be standing holding the walker. Decorate it with things that will appeal to them, encouraging curiosity and engagement. Make it a fashion statement. You could use flowers and photos of family members for a woman or stud it out Harley style for a man. Jack it up! Attempt to make the assistive devise a desire rather than an obstacle.

Exercise

Name four serious safety concerns for people with cognitive issues.

1. _____

2. _____

3. _____

4. _____

How can I help prevent a wandering person from exiting?

_____

_____

_____

_____

What can I do to help prevent a fire?

_____

_____

_____

_____

What are some dangerous items I should lock up or remove from the home?

_____

_____

_____

_____

What are two ways to approach the conversation about giving up driving that comes from a place of love?

1. _____

2. _____

Name three alternative modes of transportation for your loved one.

1. _____

2. _____

3. _____

Reflection

It's not a matter of "IF" they will do something dangerous, it's a matter of "WHEN!"

Don't be a statistic!

CHAPTER 10

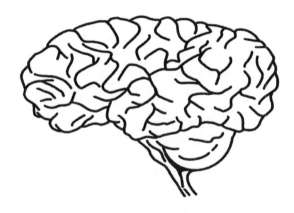

THE END, EXPLAINED
IN PLAIN ENGLISH

The Final Chapter-Death and Dying

Forget Me Not

This Chapter Has Been Omitted

At the last minute, I have decided to omit this chapter. I wanted to dedicate this book to creating a better quality of life for the living. When I began my journey, the goal was to share my infinite knowledge about caring for those with Alzheimer's or other dementias. My deep desire is to help as many families and professionals as possible.

Those with dementia need and deserve to be surrounded by people who have the necessary skills to navigate through this incredibly difficult time. And caregivers deserve access to top-notch insight and training to best care for those suffering from this debilitating disease.

I am often asked: How does a person with dementia pass away? What will it be like? So, although this chapter has been omitted, it was written, and you can access it, free of charge, by going to my website at **www. AnswersAboutAlz.org.**

If you felt that the information in the book has been helpful, please let me know!

I would also love to hear your stories. Share with me the good, the bad, and the ugly. Who knows, maybe you'll be in the next book!

Email me at <u>Debra@AnswersAboutAlz.org</u>.

ABOUT THE AUTHOR

Debra Kostiw gets fired up about advocating for seniors. Her passion ignited over a decade ago with the simultaneous opening of her home care business and her mother's diagnosis of Alzheimer's disease. Kostiw is now transforming the way we look at cognitive care through the organization she founded, Answers About Alzheimer's, Inc.

Debra's mother was manipulated into signing a Power of Attorney and moved to another state, where she was physically, financially, and psychologically abused for two and a half years, until her predator took her precious life (view Debra's full story on YouTube and www.AnswersAboutAlz.org). It was this devastating tragedy that influenced Kostiw to fight tirelessly for all seniors. Kostiw's first law, which would prevent someone from inheriting money if convicted of elder abuse, is currently on the floor of the New York State Senate.

Solicited by the Alzheimer's Association to educate the medical community and approached by WYSL to host her own radio show, Debra Kostiw is an influential Alzheimer's and dementia trainer pioneering new models for dementia care. Her life's work is devoted to those with cognitive decline and a desire to inspire a stronger, broader awareness of elder abuse.

ABOUT THE ILLUSTRATOR

Olivia Kostiw is on her way to a successful career in the arts. Olivia has professionally designed several book covers and is debuting her talents as an illustrator for Forget Me Not. Among other things, Kostiw creates one-of-a-kind gemstone jewelry. You can purchase one of her beautiful creations on the Depop App: https://depop.com/livkos2 or search her handle @LivKos2

Learn from an Industry Leader
World-Class Engaging Content

Debra Kostiw is an experienced, energetic public speaker and corporate trainer, with specific focus on topics relating to senior living communities, home care agencies, hospitals, and memory care centers. Wherever the venue, Debra succeeds in getting the audience engaged through her passion, energy and connectivity. For information about booking Debra for your next corporate training or public speaking event, or to inquire about one-on-one training, please contact: Info@AnswersAboutAlz.org

If you are interested in bulk orders of *Forget Me Not*, you may inquire at the same email address. Please identify whether you would like paperback or hardcover and the total quantity.

More information about Debra and *Forget Me Not* is always available on her website: www.AnswersAboutAlz.org

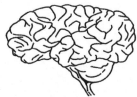

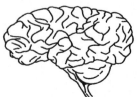

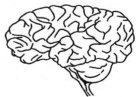

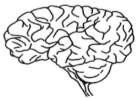

_____

_____

_____

_____

_____

_____

_____

_____

_____

_____

_____

_____

_____

_____

_____

_____

_____

_____

_____

_____

_____

_____

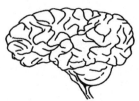

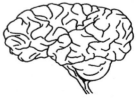

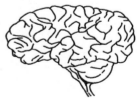

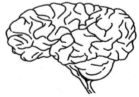

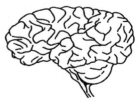

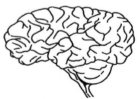

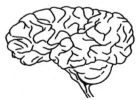

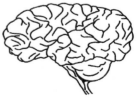

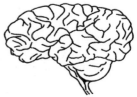

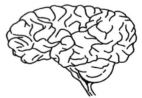

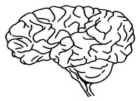

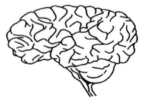

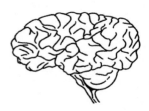

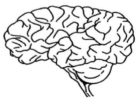

Printed in Great Britain
by Amazon

36234577R00106